Research Methodology and Its Application to Nursing

Research Methodology and Its Application to Nursing

Edited by

YVONNE M. WILLIAMSON, R.N., M.P.H., Sc.D.
Formerly Assistant Professor
The Johns Hopkins University
School of Health Services
Baltimore, Maryland

A WILEY MEDICAL PUBLICATION
JOHN WILEY & SONS
New York • Chichester • Brisbane • Toronto

Library of Congress Cataloging in Publication Data:
Main entry under title:

Research methodology and its application to nursing.

(A Wiley medical publication)
Bibliography: p.
Includes index.
1. Nursing—Research. I. Williamson, Yvonne M.
[DNLM: 1. Nursing. 2. Research—Methods.
WY20.5 R432]
RT81.5.R463 610.73'072 80-22919
ISBN 0-471-03313-8

Printed in the United States of America

10 9 8 7 6 5 4 3 2 1

This book is dedicated to my nursing research students, who deserve a standing ovation for their great interest in nursing research and for their outstanding ability to gain new knowledge in this exciting field.

Contributors

Cheryl S. Alexander, R.N., Ph.D., is an Assistant Professor in the graduate school of The Johns Hopkins University School of Hygiene and Public Health, Baltimore, Maryland, with teaching and clinical experience in maternal-child health and psychiatric nursing. She has published articles and given presentations on such topics as rape victims, the use of vignettes in survey research, and job satisfaction among hospital nurses.

Gina Bohn Browne, R.N., Ph.D., is an Associate Professor in the graduate nursing program at McMasters University, Ontario, Canada. Her nursing and social psychology experiences have been in service settings, and she has many publications and professional presentations to her credit on such social psychology topics as nursing in a primary care setting and nursing diagnoses and patient outcomes.

Norma J. Christman, R.N., M.S.N., formerly a doctoral candidate and Assistant Professor in the undergraduate program of the College of Nursing, Wayne State University, Detroit, Michigan, is currently on the faculty of The University of Arizona College of Nursing, Tucson, Arizona. She has researched and published articles on the nursing process and on the clinical performance of baccalaureate students.

Sandra J. Eyres, R.N., Ph.D., is an Associate Professor in the graduate program in maternal-child health at the University of Washington, Seattle, and Director of Nursing Research Facilitation Office at that university. She has taught research methods and has done research in public health. She has published a large number of articles on evaluative research and is presently writing a book on the nursing care in HMOs.

Phyllis Giovannetti, R.N., B.N., is a doctoral candidate at The Johns Hopkins University, Baltimore, Maryland. She has had experience in teaching, clinical nursing, and research and has published articles on patient classification systems and nurse staffing patterns.

Jean E. Johnson, R.N., Ph.D., is Professor and Chief of Oncology and Associate Medical Director of Nursing in the Cancer Center at the University of Rochester, Rochester, New York. She has had extensive teaching and clinical nursing experience and has published a large number of articles on social psychology and cancer.

Ruth M. Pallister, R.N., M.N., is an Assistant Professor at McMasters University, Ontario, Canada, in the undergraduate nursing program. In addition to teaching and consulting, she has published papers on child psychiatric nursing.

Caroline M. White, R.N., Dr.P.H., is an Associate Professor, University of Maryland, Baltimore, in the graduate program in community health nursing. She has had experience in education, administration, and research, and she has published and given presentations on community health nursing.

Yvonne M. Williamson, R.N., M.P.H., Sc.D., was Assistant Professor at The Johns Hopkins University, Baltimore, Maryland, in the undergraduate nursing program from 1976 through 1977. Before that, she lectured on research methods and statistics to undergraduates, and provided research seminars to graduate students at the University of Maryland School of Nursing. She has had nearly twenty years' experience in nursing practice and research, was a consultant for the World Health Organization (WHO) and Incarnate Word College, and has published several articles.

Preface

Nursing research is more important today than ever before, for better patient care, improved levels of health, and the future of nursing. Nurses, as the single largest category of health care providers, work throughout our complex health care system with individuals, families, groups, and communities in all phases of health and illness. Nurses participate in every aspect of health care. Because of this comprehensive involvement with patients, nurses bring a special perspective to research. Consequently, they should continue to expand their research efforts to understand what constitutes effective nursing practice and how to achieve it.

Nurses are engaging in research because they realize that significant nursing contributions to health must be based on research foundations. The challenges facing nurse researchers are formidable, given the difficulty of isolating causal relationships in the complex, interactive system of health care. Opportunities to use true experimental designs are rare, thus underscoring the need for innovative approaches. As difficult as these problems may be, achieving effective and efficient nursing care cannot be left to chance alone. Nurses must actively promote it by studying and conducting nursing research and utilizing research findings.

This book provides a comprehensive overview of the entire research process. It was written primarily for baccalaureate nursing students, but it can also be used by beginning graduate students in nursing and by professional nurses not presently engaged in formal educational programs. Although several other nursing research texts discuss the research process, none is comprehensive for baccalaureate-level nursing students. For example, some texts focus on theoretical frameworks underlying research questions but give little attention to the application process; others fail to provide the material needed to analyze data. Some texts are not logically organized in accordance with the research process; others fail to emphasize such major aspects of research as ethics and critiquing. *Research Methodology and Its Application to Nursing* is a fundamental research text that articulates the relationship between applied nursing theories, research, and practice. It provides, in logical sequence, the material needed to conduct a research study.

Because I am committed to the belief that nurses should be critical consumers of nursing research as well as competent participants, the book is organized around the various phases of an investigation. It prepares students to identify pertinent research questions, to explore relevant theories and concepts, to state the research question in a manner amenable to testing, to select and implement a study design, and then to analyze and present findings concisely. It also emphasizes the knowledge and skills needed to critique research reports. This ability should enrich students' practice as well as their research.

My objectives in editing and writing this text were several: first, to help guide and direct a core of nurses into the research field; second, to provide nurses with the knowledge and skills needed to evaluate critically the research efforts of others, especially regarding the relevance of research findings to their own practice; third, to help nurses participate effectively and comfortably in research projects that may be conducted in their work settings; fourth, to strengthen nurses' awareness of their role in protecting the rights of participants in research projects and their sense of professional responsibility for seeking out and implementing relevant research findings. Finally, it is my hope that this book will encourage nurses to develop and actively support nursing research programs.

Y. M. W.

Acknowledgments

I wish to thank my parents, Dr. and Mrs. C. Vernon Williamson, my daughter Ann, and my dear friend, Dr. Kay B. Partridge, for their continued interest, enthusiasm, and encouragement toward the completion of this book. They helped make its development possible, pleasant, and fun. Also, I would like to express my sincere appreciation to my former advisor, Dr. Philip D. Bonnet (formerly of The Johns Hopkins University School of Hygiene and Public Health) and to many professional friends, especially Marian D. McGee, Dr.P.H., Maureen C. Maguire, M.S.N., and Dorothy L. Gordon, D.Sc.N. for their careful reading of the manuscript and valuable suggestions. The contributing authors are experts in their fields, and I would like to acknowledge their scholarly and well-written chapters. Lastly, my editor, Cathy Somer, was especially supportive and knowledgeable in helping me to reach the goal of publishing this book. I am most grateful.

Y. M. W.

Contents

Research Methodology
and Its Application
to Nursing

Part 1

INTRODUCTION TO RESEARCH

Part 1 of this book presents the foundation for the research process. The importance of research in nursing is explained in Chapter 1, and the ethical issues about which student nurse researchers must be concerned are discussed in Chapter 2. The first chapter introduces the student to the value of theory and research in building a scientific foundation for nursing practice. The roles of models, conceptual frameworks, and theoretical frameworks are explained, and examples are given. Chapter 2 stresses the importance of following proper ethical guidelines in conducting research. Special emphasis is placed on the guidelines published by the federal government, the issues of informed and proxy consents, and the nurse's responsibility in clinical practice or on teaching faculties to protect the rights of human subjects participating in biomedical and behavioral research. This chapter gives examples of past as well as present research to show the student the relevance of research to nursing.

1 The Importance of Research in Nursing

Norma J. Christman
Jean E. Johnson

Why is research important to nursing? People upon whom society bestows the status of professionals are expected to be self-directing in their functions and accountable for the results of their actions on clients. In order to be self-directing, professionals must acquire knowledge relevant to the decisions they make about actions to be taken. Professionals draw on many sources of information, put information together in unique ways, and make decisions about problems. Much of the knowledge that nurses use in their decision making process is tentative—what is true today may be rejected in the future. If the profession did not include members engaged in testing and evaluating the truth of the knowledge used by the profession, the knowledge base would soon become obsolete. The practice of the profession would fail to meet its goals. Nursing would no longer be viewed as capable of meeting its responsibilities to society. For nursing to maintain its status as a profession, its knowledge base must constantly be questioned and expanded. Research is an important way to achieve that goal.

Why should the research process be included in nursing education programs? Are all nurses responsible for refuting existing knowledge and advancing new knowledge to take its place? Courses that introduce the research process are not intended to prepare people to conduct the sophisticated work required to advance scientific knowledge. The purpose of such courses is to acquaint students with the nature of the scientific process, to allow them to gain a realistic appreciation for the type of knowledge that the process produces, and to increase their ability to use that knowledge as they practice nursing. When practicing nurses have an appreciation for the contributions of research to their functions and the ability to use the knowledge research generates, there is a need for some members of the profession to acquire the advanced training necessary to learn the skills required to create new knowledge. With the researcher generating knowledge and the practitioner using that knowledge the goals of the nursing profession can better be achieved.

An appreciation of the components of the process of generating and testing knowledge is necessary before the products of such work can appropriately be used by nurses in their practice. Effective practice requires selection of relevant knowledge and evaluation of the usefulness of the knowledge in a specific situation. The process of generating knowledge often places limitations on how generally the knowledge can be applied. For example, a method of delivering care found to be effective in a large hospital may not be effective in a small hospital. The large hospital may have different characteristics such as degree of illness or socioeconomic status. The problem of treatment of decubitus ulcers provides another example that illustrates the importance of understanding how knowledge is generated when making decisions about care. Before using a method to treat a decubitus ulcer that was reported to be effective, a nurse should compare study subjects and the specific client or concern on such factors as nutritional and neurologic status.

When nurses understand the purpose of the components of the research process, they can evaluate contributions to knowledge from research and be discriminating in the use of that knowledge. Knowledge generated through research activities should not be indiscriminately accepted as "truth." Universal truths are rare. Understanding the purpose of the research process provides the means for making judgments about the usefulness of the knowledge generated by research. One need not indiscriminately accept or reject such contributions to knowledge.

Perhaps the most important thing to be gained from learning about the research process is the freedom to question in constructive ways existing practices and knowledge. If questioning or doubting leads to insecurity and lack of confidence in one's ability to practice as a nurse, it is destructive. If questioning stimulates thinking about problems in new ways and in seeking additional information, it is constructive and increases the nurse's confidence in her or his ability to practice. Nurses who ask questions about the things they do and seek answers to those questions will not only use new knowledge as it is generated, but will also stimulate the development of knowledge needed by nursing to advance the quality of care the public receives.

Learning to question in a constructive way is not easy. It is even more difficult to learn to question if one has been socialized into a system that does not value such behaviors. Therefore, nurses should be helped to learn to question early in their educational programs and should continue to develop that ability throughout their careers. Some nurses will be especially intrigued by the process of asking questions and finding answers. These nurses will elect to study in depth the process by which knowledge is developed by earning advanced degrees and becoming researchers and scientists in the nursing profession.

THE NATURE OF KNOWLEDGE

The knowledge upon which nursing, as well as other professions, bases its practice has several sources. Knowledge may be defined as the sum of what is known. Cohen and Nagel (1934) have identified four ways of knowing. First is the method of tenacity, in which knowing is based on habit, and contradictory evidence is blocked from awareness. The second way of knowing is the method of authority. By this method people appeal to respected or revered sources as a means of upholding their viewpoints. Intuition, self-evident knowing, is the third method. The fourth method of knowing is that of science or reflective inquiry that produces scientific knowledge. All four ways of knowing are used in the practice of nursing.

Research is considered by some people to be limited to the generation of scientific knowledge. Although research is the cornerstone of that way of knowing, methods of systematic investigation are relevant to the other types of knowledge. When the answer to the question "Why do you do it that way(?)" is "Because I have always done it that way," the person is basing action on habit. Such behaviors can be questioned and challenged with a systematic collection of facts. The effectiveness of such habitual behaviors might be determined by collecting data about the cost in time and money as well as the effects of the method on the client. Then these data could be compared to data obtained using an alternative method. For example, a comparison of methods of obtaining urine samples could be made by collecting data about the amount of time required to obtain a sample, the amount of contaminants in the urine, and the acceptability of the method to the client. The data from the investigation could be used to help persuade nurses to adopt the method that was found to be the most efficient, effective, and acceptable. A habitual behavior would be replaced and the new behavior would then become a habit; however, the new habitual behavior would be based on an understanding of why it is being done.

There is an area of research called policy research that is relevant to the method of knowing by authority because policy is an authoritative statement. Policy research involves analyzing and predicting the effects of principles that are used to guide decisions. Policy research uses knowledge generated by the methods of scientific inquiry instead of generating that type of knowledge.

Knowing by intuition has a special relationship to scientific knowledge. When people know something intuitively, they often know more than they realize. Some of the important discoveries in science resulted from the investigation of hunches or intuitively knowing. Intuition and creativity can be closely linked. Creative and different ways of thinking about problems lead to asking new questions, finding answers, and developing scientific knowledge.

Scientific knowledge is a unique way of knowing because it can be developed only by the methods of research or science. It has characteristics that help to define it as a distinctive way of knowing (Nagel, 1961). Science seeks to explain the relationships that exist between factors; it seeks to answer the question of *why* certain factors coexist and *explain the nature* of their coexistence. More specifically, science searches to identify when one factor is caused by another and to identify when one factor is related in a particular way to the presence of a second factor. In other words, science explains through establishing whether the relationships between factors are causative or associational.

The two basic types of relationships are illustrated in the following example: science has established that specific bacteria, one factor, cause specific infectious processes, a second factor (the tubercle bacillus causes tuberculosis). Science has also established that poor nutrition, a third factor, is associated with a higher incidence of tuberculosis; however, poor nutrition does not cause tuberculosis.

Through establishing the nature of relationships between factors and how other factors affect these relationships, science also establishes parameters, or boundaries, within which the knowledge holds. Using the previous example of tuberculosis, science has determined the relationships that exist between the tubercle bacillus, the presence of poor nutrition, and the incidence of tuberculosis as it varies with living conditions. Due to the mode of transmission of the tubercle bacillus, the incidence of tuberculosis is higher in crowded living conditions than it is in uncrowded conditions. Thus, although the relationship between the tubercle bacillus and tuberculosis is the same in all population groups, and its boundaries are universal, the probability of this basic relationship will vary with the presence or absence of other factors (specifically nutritional status and living conditions). Identification of these factors and how they are related to the basic one between bacteria and infection establishes the boundaries for use of this particular segment of scientific knowledge.

Scientific knowledge is further characterized by the logical nature of the relationships it specifies. Rules of logic are used to eliminate inconsistencies or contradictory explanations.

It is the nature of scientific knowledge to be more tentative than other types of knowledge. Because people hold onto their habits and views, authoritative ways of knowing tend to be more enduring over time. But because the scientific method generates knowledge in which the nature of the subject under study is clearly defined, there is a chance of the knowledge being refuted. Consider the possibility of refuting a statement about human beings in general, such as it is human nature to be inherently good, versus refuting the statement that some people possess the Type A coronary prone behavior pattern. The latter is much less vague and more specifically defined. Therefore, data can be collected and the existence of this particular personality type can be established or refuted.

Finally, scientific knowledge is repeatedly challenged by reexamination of the data that was gathered using controlled techniques and conditions. The techniques and conditions also are subjected to careful scrutiny. Such reexamination ensures that the specific methods used were adequate to support the claim that knowledge has been generated. If questions are raised as a result of reexamination of the data or concern is expressed about the appropriateness of the techniques and conditions of the inquiry, the validity of the scientific knowledge becomes questionable. Alternative propositions may be offered and subsequently tested. New methods of testing the original proposition may be tried and perhaps the proposition will be accepted. In that case the proposition was always true, but the methods used to test it were not adequate. It is in this manner that scientific knowledge advances.

In summary, the characteristics of scientific knowledge are dependent upon the testability of assertions about the nature of relationships between factors. Propositions that are potentially refutable through use of the methods of scientific inquiry are the only means of advancing scientific knowledge (Popper, 1968). Theory, an interrelated set of propositions that presents an explanation of the relationships between the factors that make up a particular phenomenon, is not truly theory until it has been subjected to attempts at falsification and has withstood those tests. Even then, scientific knowledge or theory remains tentative; new and different tests may alter or expand the current state of knowledge. The theory as altered by the new assertion is once again subjected to systematic investigation. Science as a way of generating knowledge is cyclic and dynamic; its product is constantly in a state of flux. Yet, it represents the best of our abilities to know and understand the varied phenomena that exist in our constantly changing and complex world.

AN EXAMPLE OF THE ADVANCEMENT OF SCIENTIFIC KNOWLEDGE

In the 1950s Janis (1958) proposed that a patient's ability to cope with the experience of surgery was related to his or her level of preoperative fear. The relationship between preoperative fear and coping following surgery was proposed to be curvilinear. Janis asserted that patients who exhibited moderate levels of preoperative fear coped better during the postoperative period than did patients who experienced either low or high levels of preoperative fear. He presented data gathered through observations and interviews with patients who were undergoing a variety of surgical procedures that ranged in extensiveness from a herniorrhaphy to intraperitoneal and intrathoracic procedures. The descriptive data he reported supported the notion that those patients who experienced moderate levels of preoperative fear also experienced less negative emotional disturbances, anger, depression, and hostility, during their postoperative course than did patients who evidenced either low or high levels of preoperative fear.

Janis' basic theoretic position concerning the nature of fear was derived from Freudian theory in which fear and anxiety serve as a drive for subsequent behavior. From this theoretic position it may be deduced that patients with low fear should be made more frightened to stimulate them to worry, that those with high fear would benefit from reduction of their negative emotional state so that their worry would be productive, and that those with moderate fear had an appropriate level of arousal to stimulate worry.

In the ensuing years, other scientists began to question Janis' theoretic position as well as the validity of the relationships his data presented. There arose an alternative view of the nature of emotion. Scientists proposed that emotion was not a drive, a compelling action, but was a response that occurred as a result of a person's assessment of his personal and environmental resources for dealing with a harmful or stressful situation (Lazarus, 1968, 1974). Further, emotion was viewed as potentially independent of behavior; that is, emotion does not inhibit action in all situations (Leventhal, 1970). Scientists, viewing emotion as a response, also questioned whether a patient's emotional response to an impending herniorrhaphy would be the same as that of a patient who was about to undergo intrathoracic surgery because of the realistic differences in threat to life posed by these operations. Thus, these scientists questioned the validity of the relationship identified by Janis because of an aspect of the scientific method he employed. In essence, they argued that a better test of the relationship between preoperative fear and postoperative coping would be achieved by limiting the study to patients who all had the same type of surgical procedure. In that way they controlled for factors that were not relevant to the theory but could influence the fears of patients.

Two studies limited to patients having abdominal surgery sought to clarify further the relationship between preoperative fear and postoperative negative emotions (Johnson, Leventhal, and Dabbs, 1971; Sime, 1976). Both of these studies failed to support Janis' theory. Patients who experienced low preoperative fear were found to experience low postoperative negative emotions such as anger, depression, and hostility. Patients whose preoperative fear was moderate experienced moderate amounts of negative moods postoperatively, and patients who were very frightened preoperatively experienced high amounts of negative moods during the postoperative period. Postoperative emotion was directly (linearly) related to the degree of preoperative emotion. Thus, neither of these studies supported Janis' proposition that patients with moderate preoperative fear will evidence the best postoperative adjustment.

Another study based on Janis' theoretic position tested the effect of providing information about surgery in an attempt to stimulate preoperative fear and thereby decrease postoperative negative emotions (Vernon and Bigelow, 1974). Information concerning surgery did not stimulate an increase in preoperative fear as predicted. Neither was postoperative negative emotion related to preoperative emotional state in this study. Once again the relationship between preoperative fear and postoperative emotion as proposed by Janis was not supported.

These research studies illustrate how alternative propositions concerning the nature of the relationship between factors stimulate systematic investigation of the originally proposed relationship as well as study of the alternative proposition. Scientific knowledge is advanced whether the original or the alternative proposition is supported. Had Janis' position been upheld, knowledge would have been advanced because his position was supported by use of methods of inquiry that involved more scientific rigor. However, as discussed above, scientific knowledge was advanced through systematic inquiry that supported an alternative view of the nature of fear before surgery and the relationship between pre- and postoperative emotional states. Scientific knowledge concerning the relationship between pre- and postoperative emotional states will continue to advance as exploration of the nature of emotional response to surgery and to other stressful situations continues. Such inquiry will help to clarify the boundaries or circumstances under which the proposed relationship occurs.

THEORY, RESEARCH, AND SCIENTIFIC KNOWLEDGE—A REVIEW

From the preceding discussion it should be evident that the characteristics of scientific knowledge are derived from its two separate but interrelated components, theory and research. To clarify the role that each of these components plays in the development of scientific knowledge, they will be briefly defined and discussed below.

Theory may generally be defined as a set of interrelated statements that provide a representation of the structure and form of a particular segment of the observable world (Dubin, 1969). Through these statements, theory specifies and defines the components of the phenomenon of concern. The components are called concepts. By describing how the various concepts that comprise the phenomenon are related, theory also provides an explanation of the phenomenon. These statements are called propositions. Through providing a description of the concepts and an explanation of the relations among them, theory enables prediction. Once subjected to confirmation through systematic investigation, theory may guide understanding of, and judgment about, the particular phenomenon with which the theory deals. At this point theory becomes scientific knowledge.

Research, a set of exacting methods and procedures, permits critical examination of the propositions set forth by a theory. Through these methods and procedures the propositions are subjected to tests to determine whether they mirror reality, the observable world. Samples of the concepts specified by the theory are obtained from the real world and examined to see if they are indeed related as proposed by the propositions. Once subjected to the methods of research and subsequently supported by these methods and their findings, theory becomes scientific knowledge useful in understanding and making decisions about the phenomenon of concern. Research findings that do not support the theoretic propositions may be used to revise the theoretic structure. Retesting and revision of the theoretic propositions may continue until they are found to mirror the real world or to be of no value.

Together theory and research constitute the process of scientific inquiry which leads to the advancement of scientific knowledge. Chapters 4 through 6 provide a detailed discussion of theory and the development of testable propositions. The methods of research that allow tests of the propositions are discussed in Chapters 7 through 14. Finally, Chapter 15 presents methods of critiquing and reporting research findings.

KNOWLEDGE, RESEARCH, AND NURSING AS A PROFESSION

Adherence to the service ideal is the major characteristic of a profession. Concern for the client is placed above concern for the professional person and the profession as a whole. As introduced earlier, a profession is characterized by the possession of a systematized knowledge base that its members use in providing service to the public. Additional characteristics of a profession are directly derived from its claim to a particular knowledge base (Wilensky, 1964).

Because of its systematized knowledge, a profession maintains exclusive jurisdiction over an area of service to the public. A specific knowledge base enables the members of a profession to provide a service to the public that cannot be obtained from someone without that particular knowledge base. Possession of specialized knowledge that enables service also allows the profession to maintain a certain degree of autonomy. Entry into a profession is dependent upon attaining the profession's base of current knowledge; therefore, a profession sets standards for the entrance and education of its new members. Professions also establish codes of ethics that set guidelines by which their members are expected to make use of the knowledge in providing service to the public. Thus, a profession's knowledge base becomes the pivotal factor that enables it to meet its primary goal, service to the public. The profession's sphere of knowledge also forms the basis from which the group maintains its professional autonomy, its authority and freedom in self-regulation and function within its area of knowledge based competence.

A group's claim to professional status and its autonomy may be threatened when its knowledge base is either too broad and vague or too narrow and restricted (Wilensky, 1964). A broad and vague knowledge base may inhibit the public's ability to identify and value the service provided by the group. Under these circumstances it may be difficult to determine how the service provided by one group differs from that of another group. On the other hand, a narrow and restricted knowledge base may be so specific that it is readily learned by the general public. Therefore, need for the group's service may be limited or nonexistent.

Nursing's professional status may be viewed as suffering from possession of a knowledge base that is quite broad and in many instances vaguely defined. The knowledge base for nursing, as it exists today, has been broadly drawn from the biologic and social sciences, physiology, chemistry, physics, sociology, psychology, and so forth. Nursing's knowledge base may be viewed as vague because it frequently does not clearly define how the knowledge from other disciplines is particularly useful in assisting people to maintain or regain their health. For example, knowledge drawn from the discipline of psychology about the development and maintenance of one's self-concept throughout the life cycle is considered relevant to nursing. Nursing textbooks propose that illness and health care activities may alter an individual's self-concept and also offer specific nursing activities to assess the degree of the impact of illness on self-concept. These textbooks assist the person in maintaining or regaining his or her self-concept. As in this example, the use of knowledge from other disciplines is generally characterized by a combination of intuitive and untested reasoning. In other words, nursing knowledge has originated more from the methods of intuition, authority, and habit than it has from the method of science.

The method of science provides the means for nursing to generate a knowledge base that is less broad and vague and, in the process, to facilitate the further development of nursing as a profession. From the above example of the use of knowledge about self-concept, research as a component of the method of science might address such concerns as: 1) the specific effect of a chronic illness on a person's self-concept; 2) whether acute and chronic illnesses differ in their impact on people's self-concept; 3) the relationship between self-concept and coping with illness; and 4) the identification of specific methods to support and maintain self-concept in situations of deviation from health. Research resulting from intellectual reasoning about the nature of a person's self-concept, tests to determine how illness affects self-concept, tests of propositions about the relationship between self-concept and health, and tests of methods to promote maintenance or restoration of self-concept, could generate knowledge that is less vaguely defined and more specifically related to the goal of the nursing profession.

Systematic inquiry similar to that suggested above draws on existing knowledge to generate new knowledge that is more specifically relevant to the purpose of nursing. Such inquiry has been and is presently being carried out by scholars in nursing. Such activity will gradually define more clearly nursing's body of knowledge, increase its professional status, and thereby increase nursing's ability to serve the public.

THE DEVELOPMENT OF NURSING KNOWLEDGE—A HISTORICAL OVERVIEW

The current state of nursing's knowledge base being the product of nursing's history is a truism which may at first seem trite and obvious. Yet, a knowledge of the facts of history, and an appreciation of their impact on the profession, are crucial to the understanding and significance of the status of nursing's scientific knowledge base. Reviewing nursing's history helps to explain the present and provides guidance for the future. From the profession's history, one may gain an appreciation of nursing's accomplishments as well as identify those factors that have impeded the development of a scientific knowledge base. Such understanding underscores the importance of past as well as present and future activities aimed at scientific inquiry in nursing.

The modern nursing profession's origin in the work and efforts of Florence Nightingale represents an equivocal picture of the use of scientific inquiry. Examination of Nightingale's interests and contributions reveals a strong commitment to the use of systematic investigation. But, on the other hand, she did not advocate the type of training and education for nurses that leads to scientific inquiry. She used the methods of systematic data collection, statistical analysis, and presentation to argue for, and to acquire, improved health care for the public. She is well known for her use of that method to illustrate the plight of British soldiers in the Crimea and India, and to persuasively argue for improved services and sanitary conditions for those soldiers (Palmer, 1977). Because of her use of statistics in the analysis of the data she collected, Florence Nightingale was recognized for her contributions to the field of statistics by the statistical societies of both England and the United States (Grier and Grier, 1978).

Even though Nightingale herself was well educated, a particularly unusual feat for a woman in the Victorian age, she did not view liberal education as a necessary component of the preparation of nurses. With the establishment of the first modern school of nursing at St. Thomas' Hospital in London in 1860, nursing education was initiated in what was to become an apprenticeship system. Nightingale failed to recognize that her abilities and accomplishments were a function of her educational preparation; that for nurses, in general, to contribute in similar ways, they would also require a sound educational base. She viewed nursing more as a "calling" than as a profession grounded in a liberal education (Palmer, 1977).

Nightingale's contributions through the use of scientific methods were limited to the organization and delivery of health care services (Palmer, 1977; Henderson, 1964). Her pronouncements as to the functions of the nurse in caring for the sick, such as providing adequate air and light (Nightingale, 1859), were derived from experience and intuition. She did not take advantage of her ability to use methods of systematic investigation to document the effects on the courses of illnesses that were related to the nursing care activities she advocated.

With the movement of the Nightingale system of nursing education to the United States, the apprenticeship approach to the preparation of nurses proliferated rapidly. Even though the St. Thomas' Hospital school was financially and educationally independent of the hospital, few of the later schools had such independence. Hospital based and controlled schools trained their students in return for the services they provided. Students were used to meet the growing demands of the public for hospital care, and education of the student most often was a secondary concern. In these first schools, the nursing instructors were physicians. These instructors, in essence, prescribed the functions of the nurse by preparing their students to assume those duties that the physicians were willing to relinquish and felt the nurse capable of performing. Fulltime nursing instructors did not appear until after 1900 (Henderson, 1964).

In such a climate, knowing based on habit and authority became firmly entrenched in nursing. At this point there was even little use of intuitive knowing as a basis for nursing care and use of the scientific method was nonexistent. Nurses learned and did what they were taught with virtually no understanding of the scientific basis for their actions. They were not encouraged to question or to develop an inquiring attitude that is basic to the use of scientific inquiry and its product, scientific knowledge.

Thus, the preparation of nurses developed outside the usual educational system of colleges and universities in which other professions have their educational base. It was not until 1909 that the first university based program was established at the University of Minnesota. In the same year, a graduate nurse education program was also established with the opening of a Department of Nursing Education at Teachers College, Columbia University.

Even though the number of nursing schools within the general system of higher education grew over the next 50 years, hospital based nursing programs continued to predominate. It was not until 1960 that the American Nurses' Association Committee on Long-Term Goals proposed the baccalaureate degree as the basic educational preparation for professional nursing practice. Then, in 1965, the American Nurses' Association's first position paper on education for nurses was published following the House of Delegates' action supporting baccalaureate education as the basis for professional nursing practice (American Journal of Nursing, 1965).

Movement of nursing education into the system of general education was crucial to expansion of the use of scientific knowledge in nursing. With basic preparation for nursing practice within the general educational system, students of nursing were systematically able to study and acquire a foundation for practice. Opportunity to gain knowledge from the biologic and social sciences facilitated understanding of the reasons for certain nursing activities. The importance of understanding and questioning was emphasized as basic to learning, and to the practice of nursing. Students were introduced to the methods of science, and were taught to use its products. Acquisition of basic nursing education within the system of higher education also facilitated entry of nurses into higher degree programs where training for generating knowledge could be obtained through the use of scientific methods.

In spite of the fact that more nurses were prepared to use scientific knowledge between 1930 and 1960, the focus of their activities was not on the development of a systematized knowledge base for nursing practice. Demands for well-prepared and able leaders came from the fields of nursing education and nursing administration. The major concerns were with continuing to improve the quality of nursing education and the administration of nursing services. The focus of scientific inquiry was on educational systems and methods as well as on the supply and demand of nurses and how they managed patient care activities. There were only a few studies prior to 1950 that dealt with tests of specific nursing care activities (Henderson, 1964). During the 1950s awareness of the importance of scientific inquiry in nursing grew, and the first nursing journal devoted to research, *Nursing Research,* was established in 1952. By the late 1950s the focus of scientific activity began to shift toward the systematic study of nursing care activities. Since the 1960s, and particularly during the 1970s, there has been a growing concern with the development of theory in nursing and, therefore, the development of a scientific knowledge base for nursing (Gortner and Nahm, 1977).

CURRENT TRENDS IN THE DEVELOPMENT OF NURSING KNOWLEDGE

From its beginning until well into the 1960s research in nursing was viewed primarily as an end rather than as the means to an end. Research methods were used to gather facts for the purpose of describing the current state of affairs or to aid in solving problems currently concerning the profession. Review of the first 25 volumes of *Nursing Research* led Batey (1977) to conclude that the major feature of the published research that limited its ability to advance scientific knowledge was the lack of theoretical formulations to guide the investigative process. Other investigators concurred and identified the relative absence of replicative studies that would advance theory and validate knowledge. Many studies were identified as an initial step but followup activities could not be found (Barnard and Neal, 1977; Ellis, 1977; Gunter and Miller, 1977; Highriter, 1977).

With the growing emphasis on theory development, research began to be placed in its perspective as the means to an end; the development of a scientific knowledge base for nursing. Nursing scholars have become increasingly concerned with the nature of theory in general and with determining the nature of a theory that would be most important to nursing (Cleland, 1967; Dickoff and James, 1968; Hardy, 1974; Jacox, 1974; Murphy, 1971; Quint, 1967; Walker, 1971). Thus, nursing has come to recognize and value interactive components of science, theory, and research.

The increased awareness of theory, its role in the scientific method, and, therefore, its use in developing a knowledge base for nursing, has also generated several questions. Primary among these questions are: 1) Why should the nursing profession develop a theory? 2) Is nursing a basic or applied science? 3) Should nursing develop a theory of nursing, a theory for nursing, or a practice theory? and 4) What are the differences between models, conceptual frameworks, and theoretical frameworks? Each of these questions will be addressed below.

Why the Nursing Profession Should Develop a Theory

The major reason for developing a theory is its practicality. A good theory, which has been tested and supported, can be used to explain and predict what will happen in many similar situations. Instead of using isolated details and facts, knowledge of a few concepts and the relations that link them together permits one to understand and to make predictions about a specific phenomenon.

The practicality of scientific knowledge in its ability to guide actions can be illustrated by using the example of tuberculosis that was previously discussed. Knowledge of the concepts, tubercle bacillus, tuberculosis, nutrition, and living conditions, and the nature of the relationships between them permits one to explain why tuberculosis occurs and to predict those conditions under which the incidence of the illness will increase or decrease. The principles, knowledge of the relationships, have been used to guide actions. Health care workers have deduced actions to decrease the incidence of the illness by improving nutrition and altering living conditions, as well as using drug therapy to cure the illness once it occurs. Knowledge of these few concepts and their relationships has been so useful in guiding action that today the incidence of tuberculosis has been greatly decreased.

Nursing Science: Basic or Applied

Basic science generates a knowledge that explains and predicts phenomena of a fundamental nature. The origins of basic science lie in the work of such men as Galileo, Newton, and Pasteur, whose contributions to science allowed explanation and prediction of phenomena that are today considered common knowledge. Generally, basic science deals with phenomena that can be isolated, controlled, and directly observed, such as chemical reactions or bacterial growth. As such, most of what is considered basic science is generated from research conducted in either a laboratory or other contrived and controlled settings. The purpose of the research is to develop knowledge that identifies the basic elements of a phenomenon and the relationships between them, such as the chemical composition of a particular substance and how its elements combine to form the particular substance. A discipline that deals with more abstract concepts, such as roles, status, coping, or health, may be viewed by some as contributing less to basic science. The major reason seems to be that there may be less certainty that the concepts and their relationships were actually observed because they were obtained under less controlled conditions. Even so, sciences dealing with both levels of concepts contribute to the development of scientific knowledge.

Applied science is concerned primarily with prediction rather than with why prediction is possible, that is, explanation (Dubin, 1969). The applied sciences use the ability to predict from knowledge that has been generated by the basic sciences in order to develop practical applications. In other words, basic scientific knowledge is translated into activities or products that may be used in every day life or used by other members of a discipline for solving problems.

Because knowledge from other academic disciplines, such as chemistry, biology, and psychology, is used in nursing research, nursing has been referred to as an applied science. It is argued that by "borrowing" concepts from other sciences nursing's ability to develop a unique knowledge base is impeded. Such an argument fails to recognize two facts. First, knowledge once generated by a discipline becomes the property of the public and may be used for whatever purposes it serves and by any academic discipline. Second, and more important, when theory or individual concepts from another discipline are used in nursing, the theory may become altered and advanced (Hardy, 1978). Concepts from the general pool of knowledge, regardless of source, may be found to be useful in nursing because they describe and explain human behavior relevant to the restoration and maintenance of health. Before one can assume that a theory explains behavior of interest to nursing or that a concept includes behaviors in health care settings, it must be shown through research that the expectations are true. Thus, existing theory and concepts may be found to describe a part of reality that is different from that in which they were developed (Walker, 1971; Johnson, 1974).

The use of an existing theory about the nature of coping illustrates this process. Lazarus (1968, 1974) proposes that coping is the result of the cognitive processing of information about a threatening situation as well as processing of information about one's personal and environmental resources for dealing with the threat. Personal and environmental resources may include such things as usual coping mechanisms, family, and other social support systems. The degree of threat perceived by people in a particular situation is based upon their appraisal of the potential harmfulness of the situation balanced against an appraisal of their resources for dealing with the situation. When the resources are viewed as greater than the potential harm, the situation is perceived as less threatening than when the resources for dealing with it are viewed as limited.

The bulk of the research testing the relationships among personal and environmental resources and perceived threat was conducted in laboratory settings where subjects were exposed to vicarious threats, such as films of a woodworking shop accident. For these concepts to be useful in real life situations where a direct threat may occur in health care settings, the concepts must be shown to describe people's behavior in these situations. Research designed to measure a client's perception of personal and environmental resources, as well as perceived degree of threat when faced with a particular health care procedure, would provide a test of the original theory's applicability to a real life threat.

The results of these tests could confirm the relationships as proposed in the original theory. Conversely, they could lead to refinement of the original concepts and theoretic formulation. In either case, the theory could then be used to develop interventions aimed at facilitating a client's ability to cope with threatening health care situations. For example, methods to increase personal and environmental resources or to decrease the perceived degree of threat could be developed and tested to determine if they do facilitate a client's ability to cope with a particular health care event. This latter activity might be viewed by some as applied research because it is derived from the more basic knowledge about coping with threatening experiences, and deals with predicting or controlling the outcome of a client's coping with health care events.

In reality, nursing scientists are developing both basic and applied science. Some nursing scientists are focusing on the use of existing theory and its applicability to nursing. In the process, they are confirming or refining the existing theory, or creating a new theory. Other nursing scientists are focusing on linking concepts about health and nursing in new and different ways, thereby generating knowledge in this manner, while others are focusing on the development and testing of nursing interventions that have been deduced from existing scientific knowledge. Yet, there are still those who are combining these activities, who are developing and testing theories that explain and predict health behavior as well as using this knowledge to deduce and test nursing interventions.

The question of whether nursing is a basic or applied science seems less important when placed in its proper perspective. The important goal is the development of nursing knowledge that describes, explains, and allows prediction of a person's behavior in a health care situation. Such knowledge may then be used for interpreting a client's behavior and making decisions about nursing care in practice settings.

Theory of Nursing, Theory for Nursing, or Practice Theory

Concurrent with the growing emphasis on the development of nursing knowledge is debate about the nature of theory and nursing. Some nurse professionals proposed that one theory should be developed which encompasses all of the phenomena included in nursing. There were those who argued that scientific knowledge relevant to nursing will require many theories. Still, others debated whether there should be a theory of nursing or a theory for nursing (Murphy, 1971). The differentiation between a theory of nursing and a theory for nursing, is somewhat unclear. However, when the term theory *of* nursing is used, it seems to refer to an all-encompassing theory which aims to describe the nature and scope of nursing and to identify the concepts that will be included in the scientific knowledge. The team theory *for* nursing is less ambitious and aims to explain a circumscribed aspect of reality relevant to nursing. Finally, because nursing is a practice profession, others have proposed that the goal should be the development of practice theory (Dickoff and James, 1968; Dickoff, James, and Wiedenbach, 1968). The advocates of this position maintain that there is a level of theory beyond that which permits explanation and prediction. Practice theory would specify a goal for patient care and how that goal could be attained.

With regard to what the nature of nursing theory should be, evaluation of these different propositions must take into consideration the basic purpose of a theory. First, as noted previously, a theory that leads to the development of scientific knowledge must be testable. A theory is testable when representations of the concepts that are included in the theory can be directly observed in the empirical world. Further, the means of observing must be reliable and valid (the techniques used to record observations are discussed in Chapters 9 and 11). Reliability and validity are complex concepts that will be discussed in Chapter 8. It will suffice here to consider that a technique for recording observations is reliable if two observers agree on what to record, and is valid if it measures what it is intended to measure; that is, the concept. A theory of nursing that describes nursing's nature and scope would necessarily deal with concepts so abstract that the relationships among them would remain vague and untestable (Hardy, 1978). Also, as noted by Jacox (1974), no other discipline has been able to specify one unifying theory, and there is little reason to believe that nursing will be able to develop such a theory. Both Hardy and Jacox argue that nuring theory should deal with more limited, less abstract concepts, with a narrower range of reality. A theory such as this might deal with the nature of sensory deprivation, coping with health care events, or the responses of children to hospitalization. A theory dealing with a more narrow range of reality seems to be close to the notion of a theory for nursing.

Practice theory is based on the premise that knowledge which allows description, explanation, and prediction, does not adequately guide nursing practice. It is proposed that because nursing is a practice discipline, it requires a level of theory that more clearly prescribes the nature of that practice under specified conditions. Beckstrand (1978a, 1978b) cogently argues that practice theory is unnecessary because the type of knowledge which is necessary for practice, is available through the accepted methods of science when it is supported by ethical knowledge.

What will be the nature of a theory that nursing finds useful? Only the future will provide the answers. Debates about the nature of nursing theory should not expend the energies of nursing scholars, thus hindering the development of nursing knowledge. This book is concerned with what a nurse uses to evaluate and develop knowledge generated by the scientific process. Such a knowledge base is necessary to further understand the debates about the nature of nursing theory.

Models, Conceptual Frameworks, and Theoretical Frameworks

The meanings of terms such as model, conceptual framework, and theoretical framework can be confusing. The confusion about such terms may be reduced if they are related to the process of theory construction. A conceptual framework may be used in the early phase of theory construction to identify the *concepts* of concern even though the relationships among them are not clearly specified. Models are simplified representations of reality that focus on the *structure* rather than the description of the phenomenon, thereby aiding in the specification of the exact relationships among the concepts that make up the model. Finally, theoretical frameworks are those statements in which there are more precise specifications of the *concepts* and *relationships* among them (Peterson, 1977). They are more specific than conceptual frameworks and models, and permit tests of the proposed relationships that may lead to explanation and prediction of the phenomenon of concern. The term theoretical framework is often shortened to just "theory" in the sciences. Thus, each of these terms represents a different stage in the process of theory construction.

THE FUTURE

Providing nursing students with an opportunity to learn about research methods early in their studies, will create a strong force to shape the future of nursing. Nurses of the future, because of their appreciation for, and understanding of the research process, will maximize the impact of three general types of activities upon the nursing profession. These activities are: 1) documentation of the contributions of nursing to health care; 2) translation of existing knowledge into ways that can help people to achieve their health goals; and 3) creation of new knowledge.

SUMMARY

This chapter has focused primarily on the last two types of activities, but the first, documentation, is currently of concern to a large number of nurses. The current systems of providing health care are not meeting the expectations of people with respect to quality, quantity, and cost. The systems are being critically examined by the public, primarily by consumer groups and organized labor, with both state and federal governments playing major roles in the movement. The nursing profession must respond with documentation of the impact its services have on the health of the public, and with the cost of that service. Research methods are essential to the design of data-producing studies that will meet the stringent criteria for evidence of the impact and cost of the care delivered by nurses. For some time, many nurse scholars will be preoccupied with conceptualizing the health care services nurses deliver, the expected outcome of that care, and the measurement of its effects on the health and health related behavior of people. The results of such endeavors will be changes in the existing health care systems and the role of nurses in these systems. All nurses will be involved in some way in these efforts. An appreciation, by nurses, of the components and nature of the research process will increase the quality of the evidence that will influence decisions about the future of nurses in the health care delivery systems.

The translation of existing knowledge about human functions into interventions that help people achieve their health goals has just begun. This is most evident in the rapidly expanding interest in, and recognition of, the contribution of behavioral factors in health and illness. Nursing can be the major health profession in the translation of knowledge about behavior into interventions, and in administering those interventions to the public. An understanding of the process of developing scientific knowledge and theory will be as essential to practitioners who incorporate such interventions into the care system as it is to the scholars who are involved in the translation process.

When nursing practitioners have an understanding of the type of question or problem that can be investigated by using the research process, they are able to shape the efforts of the nurses with advanced research training. Members of the profession have just begun to view the problems central to nursing in a way that makes it possible to use the power of the scientific process so that solutions can be discovered. The special expertise of the practitioners and scientists of nursing is required to build the knowledge base for nursing, and to translate that knowledge into nursing interventions. Before solutions for problems of profound importance to the health of people can be found, each group of experts must share an understanding of the purposes and domain of nursing, and the research process that is essential to the creation of scientific knowledge.

BIBLIOGRAPHY

American Nurses' Association's First Position on Education for Nursing. *American Journal of Nursing,* 1965, *65,* pp. 106–111.

Barnard, K. E., & Neal, M. V. Maternal-child nursing research: a review of the past and strategies for the future. *Nursing Research,* 1977, *26,* pp. 193–200.

Batey, M. V. Conceptualization: knowledge and logic guiding empirical research. *Nursing Research,* 1977, *26,* pp. 324–329.

Beckstrand, J. The notion of a practice theory and the relationship of scientific and ethical knowledge to practice. *Research in Nursing and Health,* 1978a, *1,* pp. 131–136.

Beckstrand, J. The need for a practice theory as indicated by the knowledge used in conduct of practice. *Research in Nursing and Health,* 1978b, *1,* pp. 175–179.

Cleland, V. S. The use of existing theories. *Nursing Research,* 1967, *16,* pp. 118–121.

Cohen, M. R., & Nagel, E. *An Introduction to Logic and Scientific Method.* New York: Harcourt, Brace & World, Inc., 1934. Chapter 10.

Dickoff, J., & James, P. A theory of theories: a position paper. *Nursing Research,* 1968, *17,* pp. 197–203.

Dickoff, J., James, P., & Wiedenbach, E. Theory in a practice discipline. Part II, practice oriented research. *Nursing Research,* 1968, *17,* pp. 545–554.

Dubin, R. *Theory Building.* New York: The Free Press, 1969. Chapter 10.

Ellis, R. Fallibilities, fragments, and frames: contemplation on 25 years of research in medical-surgical nursing. *Nursing Research,* 1977, *26,* pp. 177-182.

Gortner, S. R., & Nahm, H. An overview of nursing research in the United States. *Nursing Research,* 1977, *26,* pp. 10–33.

Grier, B., & Grier, M. Contributions of a passionate statistician. *Research in Nursing and Health,* 1978, *1,* pp. 103–109.

Gunter, L. M., & Miller, J. C. Toward a nursing gerontology. *Nursing Research,* 1977, *26,* pp. 208–221.

Hardy, M. E. Theories: components, development, evaluation. *Nursing Research,* 1974, *23,* pp. 100–107.

Hardy, M. E. Perspectives on nursing theory. *Advances in Nursing Science,* 1978, *1*(1), pp. 37–48.

Henderson, V. Development of research in nursing. in L. W. Simmons & V. Henderson. *Nursing Research: A Survey and Assessment.* New York: Appleton, Century, Crofts, 1964.

Highriter, M. E. The status of community health nursing research. *Nursing Research,* 1977, *26,* pp. 183–192.

Jacox, A. Theory construction in nursing: an overview. *Nursing Research,* 1974, *23,* pp. 4–13.

Janis, I. L. *Psychological Stress.* New York: John Wiley & Sons, 1958.

Johnson, D. E. Development of theory: a requisite for nursing as a primary health profession. *Nursing Research,* 1974, *23,* pp. 372–377.

Johnson, J. E., Leventhal, H., & Dabbs, J. M., Jr. Contribution of emotion and instrumental response processes in adaptation to surgery. *Journal of Personality and Social Psychology,* 1971, *20,* pp. 55–64.

Lazarus, R. S. Emotions and adaptation: conceptual and empirical relations, in Arnold, W. J. (ed.), *Nebraska Symposium on Motivation* (Vol. 16). Lincoln: University of Nebraska Press, 1968.

Lazarus, R. S. Psychological stress and coping in adaptation and illness. *International Journal of Psychiatry in Medicine,* 1974, *5,* pp. 321–333.

Leventhal, H. Findings and theory in the study of fear communications, in Berkowitz, L. (ed.), *Advances in Experimental Social Psychology* (Vol. 5). New York: Academic Press, 1970.

Murphy, J. F. *Theoretical Issues in Professional Nursing.* New York: Appleton, Century, Crofts, 1971. Chapter 1.

Nagel, E. *The Structure of Science: Problems in the Logic of Scientific Explanation.* New York: Harcourt, Brace & World, Inc., 1961. Chapter 1.

Nightingale, F. *Notes on Nursing.* London: Harrison, 1859.

Palmer, I. S. Florence Nightingale: reformer, reactionary, researcher. *Nursing Research,* 1977, *26,* pp. 84–89.

Peterson, C. J. Questions frequently asked about the development of a conceptual framework. *Journal of Nursing Education,* 1977, *16,* pp. 22–32.

Popper, K. R. *Conjectures and Refutations: The Growth of Scientific Knowledge.* New York: Harper Torchbooks, Harper & Row, 1968.

Quint, J. C. The case for theories generated from empirical data. *Nursing Research,* 1967, *16,* pp. 109–114.

Sime, A. M. Relationship of preoperative fear, type of coping, and information received about surgery to recovery from surgery. *Journal of Personality and Social Psychology,* 1976, *34,* pp. 716–724.

Vernon, D. T., & Bigelow, D. A. Effect of information about a potentially stressful situation on responses to stress impact. *Journal of Personality and Social Psychology,* 1974, *29,* pp. 50–59.

Walker, L. O. Toward a clearer understanding of the concept of nursing theory. *Nursing Research,* 1971, *20,* pp. 428–435.

Wilensky, H. L. The professionalization of everyone? *The American Journal of Sociology,* 1964, *70,* pp. 137–158.

2
Ethics: Human Subjects in Research

Research in nursing, as in other disciplines, is rarely conducted alone. The work of research scientists invariably necessitates the involvement and support of others, including human subjects, sponsoring institutions, and research assistants. A major responsibility of nurse researchers is to demonstrate concern for the rights of others, especially human subjects. This concern should be reflected in the research questions asked, in the research design, and in the presentation of data, as well as in scrupulous attention to informed consent. Growing governmental, professional, and institutional involvement in human rights underscores how important it is for nurse researchers to be well versed in ethics, particularly the rights of individuals involved in research studies. The purpose of this chapter is to discuss major aspects of the protection of human subjects participating in research and the role of nurses in assuring that protection.

BACKGROUND

"Ethics is concerned with the rules and principles that would harmonize the aims and desires of all men . . . (Clouser, 1975, p. 387)." Ethical principles defining good and evil are the basis for codes of acceptable moral and legal behavior. They are not immutable or absolute; they change with time, perceptions, and knowledge. However, the principles change much more slowly than do their specific applications in a particular society.

The concept of ethics increasingly includes an expanding concern for the well-being of human subjects (and animals) who participate in research. The atrocities that occurred in Nazi Germany during World

War II gave dramatic impetus to movements to formally protect human subjects. The use of German Jews and other "undesirables" as subjects for experimentation and gruesome forms of "research," as well as the mass murders, led to the Nuremberg Trial after the war. Certain Nazis were held responsible for their acts which were deemed to be criminal. The Nuremberg Code of Ethics developed out of those atrocities and the succeeding trial.

In more recent years, violations of human rights can be found in universities, prisons, the military, and mental institutions. For instance, in one university it was verbally reported to this author by participants that approximately 50 female student nurses were asked to participate in a study that was designed to describe their sexual response patterns to specific male sexual overtures. These responses were observed by the research investigator. Subjects were offered financial reimbursement for their participation but were told little about the research methods. Consent to participate was gained verbally. Clearly, the psychologic risks were great for those subjects. Invasion of human rights was dramatic (Unpublished data, 1976). Precise examples of these violations are found in the "Rights of Human Beings" section of this chapter.

Since World War II, active concern for human rights, expanded to encompass all forms of research involving human beings and animals, has been evident in a continuing series of declarations, codes, and regulations. These statements are economic, social, and political, and directed toward reducing disadvantages that may occur when there are wide disparities in the power of a relationship. The United Nations developed a declaration for human rights in 1949 (Nolde, 1949) and the United States government has written regulations to ensure the protection of human subjects involved in research (Federal Register, Vol. 41, 1976). The U.N. Declaration states protection as "no one shall be subjected to torture or to cruel, inhumane or degrading treatment, or punishment (Nolde, p. 57)." Further, "no one shall be subjected to arbitrary interferences with his privacy, family, home or correspondence, nor attack upon his honor and reputation (Nolde, p. 58)." The United States government regulations ensure the protection of human subjects involved in research. These regulations include the protection of confidentiality and assurance that informed consent has been obtained and documented. Abiding by these codes and regulations protects human subjects.

Groups of health professionals and professional organizations, in addition to various governing bodies, have become concerned about human rights. Anthropologists along with other professional groups have stated that people under study must have their physical, social, and psychologic welfare protected (Bloch, Phillips and Gortner, 1977). Sociologists state that subjects in research must be protected from personal harm. They are "entitled to the rights of privacy and dignity of treatment (Toward a Code of Ethics for Sociologists, 1968, p. 318)." In addition to these codes and regulations, the American Hospital Association (Levine, 1977) developed guidelines for the conduct of research involving human subjects. A Patients' Bill of Rights (Quinn and Somers, 1974) and institutional review committees (Block, et al, 1977) have been established in most health care agencies as additional safeguards for the protection of patients.

These codes, declarations, and regulations have generally raised the status of subjects participating in research. Now researchers may no longer conduct studies without regard for the human rights of the subjects. This is true for research conducted in any institution, whether it is with patients in hospitals or nursing homes, or with students conducting research in educational settings. Nursing's involvement in research could be in the care of patients, education of students, or combinations of both.

In 1968, the American Nurses' Association first published guidelines for the nurse engaging in research (American Nurses' Association, 1968). These guidelines, updated in 1975, require that subjects must be free from risk of injury, and have their privacy and dignity protected (American Nurses' Association, 1975). The American Nurses' Association further accepted a commitment to support two sets of human rights. One set is concerned with the rights of qualified nurses (those with research preparation) to engage in research, and to have access to resources necessary for implementing scientific investigations. The other deals with the human rights of all persons who are recipients of health care services or are participants in research performed by investigators whose studies impinge on the patient care provided by nurses (American Nurses' Association, 1975, p. 1).

RIGHTS OF HUMAN BEINGS INVOLVED IN RESEARCH

Human rights are those inalienable rights of free people that are not to be withheld or impaired without their full consent. Protecting these human rights requires the researcher to be sensitive and actively responsive to the rights of others. Courtesy, regard for personal integrity, and adequate information necessary to give a fully informed consent, should be extended to human subjects. At times, the researcher will find it necessary to revise research protocols, reword questions, or alter time of data collection in order to ensure that the rights of human subjects are not abridged. The burden of adjustment and inconvenience rests with the investigator.

Violating the rights of human subjects may have serious negative consequences for everyone involved. Subjects may suffer psychologic or physical harm such as adverse drug reactions (Milgram, 1963). Also, subjects who feel that they are exploited or subjected to unnecessary risk and discomfort may bring legal action against the researcher and/or the sponsoring institution. Signed consent forms must be obtained. Less extreme reactions by subjects include refusing to participate or giving incorrect responses. Violating human rights can lead to questionable research findings, compromised professional status for the investigator, and undue administrative and legal complications for the sponsoring institutions.

Research involving human subjects is of two types: biomedic and behavioral. Biomedic research encompasses studies of human physiology or pathophysiology, such as testing the efficacy of new drugs, treatment regimens, or organ transplants (Silva, 1974). Behavioral research focuses on behavior, attitudes, knowledge, and perceptions of subjects such as satisfaction with care and the level of knowledge about diet regimen. Nursing research more often involves behavioral questions than biomedic ones.

Rights of Human Subjects in Biomedic Research

The role of human subjects in biomedic experimentation has become increasingly complex and subject to growing scrutiny. Particular attention has been focused on the special problems of research on fetuses, prisoners, and the mentally retarded and on clinical trials. This emphasis reflects the additional concern society and professionals direct toward assuring protection to those who for one reason or another are unable to enter into agreements as equals.

Although it has not always been possible, advanced technology now permits new types of research investigation of the fetus and the pregnant woman. Therapeutic research may be conducted, provided the research is reviewed by ethical review committees of the sponsoring agency. Nontherapeutic research imposes additional restraints. The fetus can be exposed only to minimal risk, if any, and it cannot be dying. Also, the investigator must show that the research will contribute important knowledge that could not be obtained in any other way. No inducement may be offered to the pregnant woman to obtain an abortion for fetal research purposes (Ingelfinger, 1977).

In the past, research on prisoners was conducted with only casual consent of the subjects. Little thought was given to implied rewards of earlier parole for participating or to implied threats for not participating in research. Prisoners might volunteer for participation in a study, hoping for parole from a long sentence for "good behavior" or "cooperation." Now such research proposals must receive consultation with a Federal ethical review body, the research must be judged by committee members to fulfill important societal and scientific needs, and it must show evidence that subjects did volunteer (Inglefinger, 1977). Although the Federal ethical review bodies state that consent must be voluntary, some observers may question whether a prisoner can act in a fully voluntary way.

People who are mentally retarded represent another group that must receive special protection in research. Gaining their informed consent is controversial. It may be difficult for the investigator to feel confident that the subject has an understanding sufficient to give his consent. Proxy consent from legal guardians may be problematic and will not necessarily guarantee safety for the subject. However, a fully informed permission from a guardian, coupled with the integrity of the investigator, is the best protection for the mentally retarded subject (Brody, 1975).

Typically, clinical trials are designed to investigate the effectiveness of different medical treatments. The research designs usually employ experimental and control groups to compare outcomes of the new methods. The control groups are those subjects who do not receive the new treatment. They receive a traditional treatment or no treatment in the form of a placebo. Thus, the control groups are denied whatever benefits may result from the new treatment. However, the control groups may also avoid any risks associated with the new treatment. This benefit/risk analysis requires undivided attention to the protection of a subject's human rights.

Rights of Human Subjects in Behavioral Research

A number of health professionals, including nurses, are particularly interested in health care behavior and the knowledge, attitudes, and perceptions associated with behavior. To obtain this information, researchers may carry out in depth observational studies with a few cases or, at the other extreme, mail survey questionnaires to a national sample of respondents. Occasionally, subjects may be exposed to distinct situations in order for different responses and reactions to be determined. Behavioral research may be directed toward the providers of care themselves so that the impact of their care can be studied. An example of provider care is seen in a study funded by a private foundation, that was designed to initiate the evaluation of an ambulatory care training program in two settings within one large urban pediatric center. A second purpose of the study was to provide input into the development of primary care education curricula. To satisfy these purposes, pediatric charts were reviewed by type of provider for 353 patients making initial visits and for 151 patients making followup visits. Charts were compared for their contents concerning health education. Provider recordings were made by Pediatric Nurse Practitioners (PNPs), hospital staff physicians and medical school faculty. Findings indicated that more PNP interactions related to the primary element of care and more physicians interactions related to diagnosis and management of patient health problems. Even though this research did not invade the biologic organism, the investigators had to be meticulous to insure that human rights were protected. Consent to conduct the research had to be gained from the institution before data were collected (Politzer, et al, 1977).

Federal Safeguards

Federal regulations require that any institution receiving federal monies to conduct research establish a committee to monitor research activities in full compliance with human rights requirements. Generally, an investigator submits a research protocol to this committee for review and approval before submitting the research proposal to the funding source (either federal or private). Specific committee functions are based on the requirements of the funding source. For the federal government, the investigator must provide assurances that human subjects are protected. The Public Health Service's *Grant Policy Statement* summarizes the policy of the Code of Federal Regulations regarding human subjects:

> Safeguarding the rights and welfare of human subjects involved in activities supported by Public Health Service grants is the responsibility of the institution that receives and is primarily accountable to the Government for the funds awarded for the support of the research, development, demonstration, or other activities that include as participants individuals who may be placed "at risk" because of their participation. An individual is at risk if he/she may be exposed to the possibility of physical, psychological, or social injury. These individuals must by protected in accordance with the provisions of the above-referenced regulation.
>
> *Title 45, CFR 46, 1976, p. 57.*

The assurance form to be completed for submission to the Department of Health and Human Resources requires specific notice if the research involves minors, fetuses, abortuses, pregnant women, prisoners, mentally retarded persons, or mentally disabled persons. This again illustrates the special attention directed to these subgroups.

INFORMED CONSENT

The principal mechanism for ensuring that individuals' rights are respected is informed consent. As practiced today, informed consent means that a person agrees, in writing, to participate as a subject in a research project, and that his decision is made with adequate knowledge of potential and real risks or benefits. Further, the subject must voluntarily give consent with the knowledge that the subject may withdraw from the study *at any time* without fear of coercion or retaliation.

The notion of informed consent is only gradually taking shape through continued use in research activities and through legal decisions. Particularly unclear is the definition of how much information is adequate to form a decision (Rutstein, 1969). Should a subject be told of *all* possible side effects of a drug, even those occurring once in 10,000 chances? How does an investigator determine the ability of a subject to weigh potential risks and benefits? How comprehensive are the written instructions? Does informing subjects in projective psychologic tests bias the responses and interpretation of the findings? How much should the subject be told about the research? Can these questions be answered by an adequate consent form (Alfidi, 1971)?

The investigator must have documentary evidence that the subject has voluntarily agreed to participate in the study with knowledge of its purposes and attendant hazards. In behavioral research, this agreement may be accomplished by the subject signing a statement that the study was verbally explained to him, that confidentiality was guaranteed, and that he agreed to participate. Further, the statement should indicate that there are minimal or no personal risks and that the subject can withdraw from the study at any time without personal repercussions. Consent for subject participation in biomedic research requires additional information. First, consent is not likely to be verbally acquired. Rather, the subject would read and sign a document that specifically indicates the study purpose, the risks involved, and any other pertinent information about his participation. This document should clearly state that the subject's response is confidential and that he has the right to withdraw at any time. The degree to which subjects are informed, in spite of these precautions, remains somewhat questionable.

Informed consent becomes even more ambiguous when consent must be obtained on behalf of the subject, as in the case of fetuses, infants, and children. An experiment on an aborted fetus may have a questionable ethical aspect. The experiment might be a violation against a fetus who is incapable of giving consent. The fetus can be used as a means for advancing a body of knowledge but not necessarily for its own benefit (McCormick, 1976). For instance, a living aborted fetus could provide important information in the continued development of diagnostic machinery such as sonography. Sonograms provide a picture of the unborn fetus by measuring its sound waves. These are no risks to the fetus or mother. This can be compared to the mother-fetal risks involved in using x-rays to obtain diagnostic pictures. Although the fetus would not necessarily benefit from this development, future fetuses and mothers may.

A more ambiguous ethical question can be seen in a current research proposal from the Institute of Embryology. In this research, the fetuses would be obtained from pregnant women who had aborted voluntarily. The fetuses then would be transferred to an artificial placenta. Ethical concerns are related to consent, especially from the religious, fetal, and the mother's perspectives (Veatch, 1977).

As seen in consent for research on a fetus, a similar problem exists in consent for research with infants and children. For instance, children are sufficiently different from adults pharmacologically, psychologically, and metabolically, to necessitate research on children in order to test drug efficacy (McCormick, 1974). Additionally, research involving infants and children is needed to further understand the development, needs, and strengths of children. A basic tenet is that regardless of the child's age, his rights supersede the rights and desires of the investigator and must be protected.

Consent for a child's participation must be obtained from parents or others legally responsible for the child. The investigator must explain all aspects of the research that may affect the child as well as answer all questions the child *and* parents have about the reasearch (Duffy, 1973). Informed permission gained from parents, as well as the integrity of the investigator, are a child's best protection from exploitation as a research subject. Opinions differ on the age at which a child may give his own consent. However, if a child is older than 14 years, his or her consent should be obtained in addition to that of the parents (Campbell, 1974).

Clearly, an important element in the concept of informed consent is that of confidentiality. Assurance must be given to the subjects that the information obtained will be kept in confidence and that no person will be identified. In the past, violating the privacy of subjects was of little apparent concern to some investigators who concentrated on gathering data with minimal attention to the possible consequences for the subjects.

Failure to consider consequences to subjects participating in research is illustrated in a famous study designed to describe destructive obedience. This study was conducted in a laboratory setting under the guise of a learning experiment, with little apparent regard for its effects on the subjects. Uninformed subjects were asked to administer electric shocks to other people participating in the study. These people were professional actors, although this fact was not divulged to the study subjects. The subjects were asked to increase the severity of the shocks when the "actors" failed to respond in the "correct" way. The "actors" were out of the subjects sight so only their groans of pain and terror could be heard. Unanticipated responses by the subjects demonstrating their destructive obedience ranged from twitching to near nervous collapse (Milgram, 1963). The human rights of these subjects were clearly violated.

Current guidelines on a patient's right to privacy and confidentiality are not limited only to research studies, but also include delivery of health services. Patient advocacy programs, established to help protect their rights, serve as a mechanism to increase the ability of patients to participate in decisions affecting their health care. The programs protect patients, for example, by providing the disadvantaged (illiterate, those alone, etc.) with the help they may need during a hospitalization. When requested by patients, the advocates represent them in addressing modern technology, and in establishing a "partnership" relationship with their physicians (Annas and Healey, 1974).

The Patients' Bill of Rights, while in a hospital and while in nursing homes, also has been developed by the American Hospital Association and published as guidelines for the rights of patients. These guidelines, posted in the hospital or nursing home facility, represent a first step on the part of health care institutions to publicly acknowledge the privileges and considerations to which patients are entitled during their stay. The statements further serve as reminders, to providers of care, of the rights of patients with respect to both patient care and research activities. In certain instances, patients are informed of what steps to take in the event they do feel their rights have been violated.

Health care facilities and educational institutions have begun to establish review committees for research in their facilitites that involves human subjects. These committees may include lay members such as lawyers, statisticians, clergy, and scientists as well as a variety of health professionals: physicians, nurses, and medical social workers (May, 1975). The purpose of such review committees is to assure responsible research and to protect human subjects from avoidable risks during the research, whether it is biomedic or behavioral. Proposals are reviewed to determine their scientific soundness and social value. Equally important, designs are evaluated to determine the risks to the subjects and the method for obtaining informed consent (Gray, 1975).

Scientific soundness in a research proposal may be determined by the relevance of the design and the consequence to the study subject. For example, in the early 1930s the Public Health Service initiated a study to test the effectiveness of mercury as a treatment for syphilis (Lasagna, 1975). The study group consisted of black male farmers over 25 years of age in Macon County, Alabama. The study was comprised of 891 subjects: 412 men with syphilis diagnosed by blood tests, 204 men without syphilis (as a control group), and 275 others who had supposedly been cured with mercury, arsenic, and bismuth. The subjects with syphilis were not treated. "All subjects in the experiment received periodic checkups and treatment for nonsyphilitic conditions as well as a yearly cash payment and burial expenses (Lasagna, p. 61)." The conduct of this study was discovered 40 years later and investigated. There was no formal research proposal, no indication of informed consent, and no treatment for the people with syphilis even though penicillin was developed and in use. It is doubtful whether this study, if reviewed today, would receive approval from human rights committees. It seems to lack ethical soundness in all regards. Human rights were not protected.

THE ROLES OF NURSES IN THE PROTECTION OF HUMAN RIGHTS

Clinical Nurses

All nurses, whether giving patient care, teaching, or conducting research, must demonstrate concern for the mental and physical safety of their patients or subjects. In the role of patient advocate, the nurse actively ensures that in all phases of health care the dignity and rights of the patient are fully protected. In addition to the obligation to protect patients, the clinical nurse involved in research would be required to consent to participate. This consent would involve certain responsibilities to the director of the research project, including keeping the director informed about current problems in the study. For example, if patient responses appeared to be unrelated to the questions asked, the nurse would inform the director and together they could diagnose the problem and plan appropriate actions. This nurse action would not only further protect the patient but also assist the director in gathering relevant data. Also it would enhance the self-confidence of the nurse participating in the study. The extent of the nurse's involvement depends, in part, upon the patient's ability to handle his own decisions. A principal function of the clinical nurse may be to listen to the patient as he explores his decision whether or not to participate. This participation may include direct involvement or an agreement to release the patient's health record to the investigator of the study. The nurse can assist by reminding the patient of his rights and prerogatives, supporting him if he desires further clarification and information, or supporting him if he wishes *not* to participate. While in certain instances a nurse may serve as a facilitator, it is the responsibility of the investigator to provide sufficient and correct information. If it is not provided, the nurse must obtain it. It is the patient's responsibility to make his own decision. The nurse should not make the decision for the patient, either directly or indirectly.

Nursing Faculties

Nursing faculties that teach research methods have a similar responsibility for the protection of human subjects. Even though faculty members may not be involved in patient care, they should oversee their students' projects with a keen concern for the rights of human subjects. This includes being informed about the ethical policies of the institution in which the research would be conducted. The faculty would need to know, for example, the institutional policies regarding the release of information on a patient's chart, the procedure for research protocol review by its ethical committee, and the steps to be taken before the onset of data collection. The nursing curriculum should include the study of ethical issues in research and patient care so that students understand the complexities and importance of this topic (Aroskar, 1977).

Nurse Researchers

Perhaps the most fundamental type of protection that can be offered by a nurse researcher to the subjects in a study is a scientifically sound research project. By involving subjects only in projects deemed by the nurse and her colleagues to be of scientific merit, she demonstrates her respect and concern for others. Hence, it is a responsibility of the nurses wishing to conduct research to acquire the requisite theoretic and practical knowledge for such investigation (*The Nurse in Research,* 1968). In addition, nurse researchers need to constantly update their information about current governmental and institutional regulations regarding human subjects, since new dimensions emerge continually.

In addition to demonstrating scientific vigor, the researcher must assiduously pursue ethical methods and procedures. This means that the framing of hypotheses, the methods of data collection, and the presentation of data, must all reflect respect for human rights. It is patently unethical to try to convince subjects that they will not be harmed or their privacy violated unless that is true. If risks exist, even potentially, those risks must be set forth in language and in a manner conducive to achieving freely given informed consent.

The reseacher must plan the study in such a way as to allow sufficient time for both the research proposal to be reviewed on behalf of human subjects and the informed consent to be meticulously obtained. Again, the researcher and all research assistants must be especially cautious to avoid pressuring subjects into participating. This goal is not always easy to achieve when dealing with people who might be easily intimidated or confused, such as children, the mentally retarded, or families of critically ill patients. Finally, presenting data only in aggregate form, never individually, will guard the confidentiality of subjects. However, special attention may, at times, need to be devoted to camouflaging institutions or towns involved in studies if guarantees of confidentiality were requested by or extended to the agency, hospital, or region. This can be achieved by using codes instead of names to identify the study subjects and sites.

These ethical concerns in research are fully consonant with the code for nurses published by the American Nurses' Association, 1976:

1. The nurse provides services with respect for human dignity and the uniqueness of the client unrestricted by considerations of social or economic status, personal attributes, or the nature of health problems.
2. The nurse safeguards the client's right to privacy by judiciously protecting information of a confidential nature.
3. The nurse acts to safeguard the client and the public when health care and safety are affected by the incompetent, unethical, or illegal practice of any person.
4. The nurse assumes responsibility and accountability for individual nursing judgments and actions.

5. The nurse maintains competence in nursing.
6. The nurse exercises informed judgment and uses individual competence and qualifications as criteria in seeking consultation, accepting responsibilities, and delegating nursing activities to others.
7. The nurse participates in activities that contribute to the ongoing development of the profession's body of knowledge.
8. The nurse participates in the profession's efforts to implement and improve standards of nursing.
9. The nurse participates in the profession's efforts to establish and maintain conditions of employment conducive to high quality nursing care.
10. The nurse participates in the profession's effort to protect the public from misinformation and misrepresentation and to maintain the integrity of nursing.
11. The nurse collaborates with members of the health professions and other citizens in promoting community and national efforts to meet the health needs of the public.

American Nurses' Association, 1976.
(Reprinted with permission.)

The nurse in any area of practice must adhere to these guidelines. Items 2, 4, and 7 are particularly relevant. Item 2 addresses the client's right to privacy in terms of disclosures of information to the health team members as well as to those not involved in the client's care. Included are disclosures in a court of law and in access to client's health records. This confidentiality ethically safeguards the client's right to privacy. Item 4, in part, states that in determining the responsibility for data collection the nurse is held accountable. Responsibility and accountability are inseparable. Finally, item 7 specifically addresses the nurse in research, giving general guidelines, protection of human rights, and the practitioner's rights and responsibilities. This code underscores the nurse's role as a patient advocate, a role that must *not* be lost when a nurse conducts research.

SUMMARY

This chapter has presented the roles of the federal government, the courts, and various professional organizations in making explicit the ethical criteria which research projects must satisfy. Attention was given to the fact that nurses can demonstrate their concern for the protection of the rights of others by keeping informed on ethical issues and implementing studies that safeguard the rights of others.

BIBLIOGRAPHY

Alfidi, R. J. Informed consent: a study of patient reaction. *Journal of the American Medical Association,* May, 24, 1971, *216* (8), pp. 1325-1329.

American Nurses' Association. *Code For Nurses With Interpretive Statements,* 1976, American Nurses' Association Publication Code No. G-56.

Annas, G. J., & Healey, J. M. The patient rights advocate. *Journal of Nursing Administration*, May/June, 1974, pp. 25-31.

Aroskar, M. A. Ethics in the nursing curriculum. *Nursing Outlook,* 1977, *25,* pp. 260-264.

Block, D., Phillips, T. P., & Gortner, S. R. Protection of human research subjects, in Miller, M. H., & Flynn, B. C. (eds.), *Current Perspectives in Nursing,* (Vol. I), St. Louis: C. V. Mosby Company, 1977. pp. 14-31.

Brody, E. B. The right to know. *Journal of Nervous and Mental Disease,* August, 1975, *161* (2), pp. 73-81.

Campell, A. G. M. Infants, children and informed consent. *British Medical Journal,* August 3, 1974, *3,* pp. 334-338.

Clouser, K. D. Medical ethics: Some uses, abuses and limitations. *New England Journal of Medicine,* August 21, 1975, *293* (8), p. 387.

Code of Ethics, by Committee of the American Sociological Association: Washington, D.C., 1968.

Committee on Ethics of the American Health Association. Ethical implications of investigations in seriously and critically ill patients. *Circulation,* December 1974, *50,* pp. 1063-1069.

Duffy, J. C. Research with children: the rights of children. *Editorial Child Psychiatry and Human Development,* Winter, 1973, *4* (2), pp. 67-70.

Federal Register, *Protection of Human Subjects.* November 30, 1976, *41* (231), Title 10, Part 745.

Gray, B. H. An assessment of institutional review committees in human experimentation. *Medical Care,* April, 1975, *13* (3), pp. 318-328.

American Nurses Association. *Human Rights Guidelines For Nurses in Clinical and Other Research,* 1975.

Ingelfinger, F. J. Ethics of human experimentation defined by a national commission. *New England Journal of Medicine,* January 6, 1977, *296,* pp. 44-45.

Lasagna, Louis. *The VD Epidemic: How It Started, Where It's Going, and What To Do About It.* Philadelphia: Temple University Press, 1975. pp. 53-72.

Levine, M.E. Nursing Ethics and The Ethical Nurse, *American Journal of Nursing,* May, 1977, *77* (5), pp 845–876.

May, W. W. The Composition and Function of Ethical Committees. *Journal of Medical Ethics,* April 1975, *1* (1), pp. 23-29.

McCormick, R. A. Proxy consent in the experimentation situation. *Perspectives in Biology and Medicine,* Autumn, 1974, pp. 2-20.

McCormick, R. A. Experimental subjects: who should they be? *Journal of the American Medical Association,* May 17, 1976, *235* (20), p. 2197.

Milgram, S. Behavioral study of obedience. *Journal of Abnormal and Social Psychology,* 1963, *67* (5), pp. 371-377.

Nolde, O. F. The United Nations Declaration of Human Rights. *Headline Series Foreign Policy Association,* July-August, 1949, *76,* pp. 55-62.

Politzer, R. M., Bledsoe, T., Morton, K. C., & Sudia, R. K. A comparison of primary care educational experiences in two urban pediatric settings. *Proceedings of the 16th Annual Conference on Research in Medical Education.* American Association of Medical Colleges, November, 1977, pp. 239-244.

Quinn, N., & Somers, A. R. The Patients' Bill of Rights. *Nursing Outlook,* April 1974, *22* (4), pp. 240-244.

Rutstein, D. D. The ethical design of human experiments. *Daedalus: Ethical Aspects of Experimentation with Human Subjects,* Spring 1969, *98* (2), pp. 523-541.

Silva, M. C. Science, ethics, and nursing. *American Journal of Nursing,* November 1974, *74* (11), pp. 2004-2007.

Stickel, D. L. Ethical and moral aspects of transplantation. *Monographs of the Surgical Sciences,* 1966, *3* (4), pp. 267-301.

The Nurse in Research: American Nurses' Association Guidelines on Ethical Values, New York; American Nurses' Association, January, 1968.

Thigpen, L. W. *Guidelines For Research In Clinical Nursing.* New York: The League Exchange Number 81, 1967.

Toward a code of ethics for sociologists. *The American Sociologist,* November, 1968, *3* (4), pp. 316-318.

Veatch, R. M. *Case Studies of Medical Ethics.* Cambridge: Harvard University Press, 1977.

Part 2

THE RESEARCH PROCESS

Part 2 presents information needed by the student to pursue research interests. Chapter 3 gives an overview of the entire research process, including types of research, types of thinking, identification of the problem, the literature review, generation of hypotheses, data gathering, data analysis, and statistics. Basic approaches to these various aspects of conducting research are discussed. Chapter 4 directs the student to theory, concepts, and nursing practice that may underlie the scientific study. In Chapter 5, the process of gathering relevant information related to a study is explained. Problem selection and hypotheses formulation are discussed in Chapter 6, which focuses on personal considerations, and social factors, and their delineations and definitions, along with operational definitions of concepts as they apply to the development of hypotheses. The development and construction of hypotheses receive special attention. Types of variables and their roles in research and null hypotheses are presented, leading to a discussion of hypotheses testing. Statistical evidence for the acceptance or rejection of hypotheses is discussed and examples are presented to illustrate each phase. After completing Parts 1 and 2, the reader is prepared to begin to consider the design of the research project.

3
Introduction to the Research Process

Gina Bohn Browne
Ruth M. Pallister

The process of scientific discovery or research is often considered to be a formidable and mysterious endeavor. Yet, every human being engages in some level of discovery and problem solving every day. The problem solving process that health professionals use daily in clinical practice is very much like the research process. Problem solving is a more informal process of identifying patient problems, exploring relationships between patient problems and other factors, observing, testing methods of treatment, and evaluating the outcomes. Research is a more formal and systematic problem solving process that attempts to minimize bias and human error.

In order to engage in disciplined enquiry, the beginning investigator must understand the terminology and steps of the research process. This chapter provides an overview of this process with the purpose of introducing the reader to the importance of systematic rigor in the conduct of any study. The steps of the research process are outlined, examples are provided, and common pitfalls at various stages are explained. Each of the steps is developed further in the remaining chapters of this book.

THE MEANING OF TYPES OF RESEARCH

There are a number of approaches to the classification of research. Research can be categorized according to:

- The type of *thinking* processes used (such as inductive or deductive thinking)

- The *depth of inquiry* carried out (exploratory, descriptive, experimental)
- The *purpose* of the inquiry itself (basic or applied)
- The *research method* and *design* used in the research process (correlational, ex post facto, etc.)

In the inductive thinking process, data are gathered in the particular category (species), and the broader category (genus) to which the species belongs is generated or conceptualized. For example, the investigator may interview a variety of patients about their concerns in the hospital and record what they say in an unstructured format. From all of the specific or individualized concerns, the investigator may identify commonalities or thematic concerns which occur in the story of almost every patient. These common or general concerns, such as fear or loss, are induced or generated from the particular data provided by each patient. This type of inductive research is often used in sociologic or anthropologic field research. The unstructured method of gathering this type of data is sometimes called participant observation. Schatzman and Strauss (1973) call this inductive approach "grounded theory," the process of "discovery" or "field research." Francis Bacon (1949) advocated this process of observation where generalizations are derived from the evidence in many individual observations. The inductive method was developed in response to the limitations of the older deductive method of thinking.

The deductive method of Aristotle (Gathrop, 1969; Organ, 1965; Whitehead, 1967) moves from the assumption, concept, or generalization (genus) to the specific application or example (species) of the generalization. For example, a knowledge based assumption is that a patient in a state of dehydration will demonstrate a rise in the specific gravity of the urine. When faced with a dehydrated patient, a nurse could predict or identify this particular outcome of a high specific gravity. The process of proposing hypotheses about relationships to be tested that are based on previous knowledge is an example of this deductive type of research.

The inductive method of Bacon (1949), with its absence of the *a priori* focus of deductive inquiry confused investigators and alone rarely led to a generalization or theory. The deductive method of Aristotle, with its potential for accepting erroneous or incomplete first assumptions, was limited without the inductive approach or verification.

Centuries later both approaches were combined in the deductive-inductive approach to research used by Darwin (Gathrop, 1969; Organ, 1965; Whitehead, 1967). This combined process can be summarized as follows:

Deductive Thinking	*Inductive Thinking*
Identification or definition of problems Formulation of an hypothesis—a hunch, assumption, or guess Organization of an approach to the collection and analysis of data	Formulation of conclusions Verification, rejection, or modification of the hypothesis originally advanced

The deductive first and second initial steps (see Deductive Thinking above) of the research process serve to focus the field of observation. The inductive steps (see Inductive Thinking above and the last item of Deductive Thinking) which follow serve to test the accuracy of the initial proposition.

This research process can be employed with varying degrees of intensity and rigor and with different purposes for the inquiry. French (1968) classified these levels of inquiry as exploratory, descriptive, or experimental. In exploratory research the investigator studies which variables or factors are relevant to a given situation. In descriptive research, the investigator studies the relationship between these factors. In experimental research, the investigator studies the effect of each variable on the other (Treece and Treece, 1977).

Any of these three levels of inquiry (research) occur in either basic or applied research. Basic research is the search for knowledge, while applied reserach tests the usefulness or applicability of this knowledge in the everyday clinical or field situation. Basic research is often called laboratory research. Applied research is often called clinical research.

Basic and applied research can be further classified according to the specific purposes and method used in either approach. Isaac and Michael (1978) offer a detailed classification of research according to the purpose and method of research used (Fig. 3-1).

In each of these broad purposes of research, the investigator undergoes similar steps of the research process as previously outlined. The remainder of this chapter offers a brief overview of each of these steps of the research process.

IDENTIFYING THE PROBLEM

The inquiring professional as well as the student nurse consider certain questions that arise in their everyday work life. For the nurse these questions may be related to or center on the:

Method	*Purpose*
Historical	To reconstruct the past objectively and accurately, often in relation to the tenability of an hypothesis.
Descriptive	To describe systematically a situation or area of interest factually and accurately.
Developmental	To investigate patterns and sequences of growth and/or change as a function of time.
Case and field	To study intensively the background, current status, and environmental interactions of a given social unit: an individual, group, institution, or community.
Correlational	To investigate the extent to which variations in one factor correspond with variations in one or more other factors based on correlation co-efficients.
Causal-comparative or ex post facto	To investigate possible cause-and-effect relationships by observing some existing consequence and searching back through the data for plausible causal factors.
True experimental	To investigate possible cause-and-effect relationships by exposing one or more experimental groups to one or more treatment conditions and comparing the results to one or more control groups not receiving the treatment (random assignment being essential).
Quasiexperimental	To approximate the conditions of the true experiment in a setting which does not allow the control and/or manipulation of all relevant variables. The researcher must clearly understand what compromises exist in the internal and external validity of his design and proceed within these limitations.
Action	To develop new skills or new approaches and to solve problems with direct application to the classroom or other applied setting.

Figure 3-1. Isaac's and Michael's nine basic methods of research. (Isaac, S., and Michael, W.B. *Handbook in Research and Evaluation.* San Diego: EdITS/ Knapp Publisher, 1971. All rights reserved. Reproduced with permission.)

- Frequency of phenomenon—how often does this occur (specify)?
- Relationship between phenomena—is this (specify) related to that (specify)?

- Cause of certain conditions—what (specify) causes this (specify) under what specific conditions?
- Cost and effect of various situations—what specific effect does this (specify) have on that (specify) at what cost (specify) with whom (specify) compared with what (specify)?

As demonstrated by these questions, the more specific, refined or well-stated the question, the easier it is to determine the method for answering the question. Experience has shown that the major proportion of research time should be spent in specifying the question (Fig. 3-2). Some common mistakes made in the research process result from skipping or sliding over the problem formulation phase.

Common mistakes made by investigators are collecting or analyzing data without a purpose, and posing a loosely stated problem without a genuine interest in the area. In evaluating the significance or relevance of a problem area before embarking on an investigation, the following questions might be asked in order to avoid usual pitfalls:

1. Are the necessary resources (tools, time, abilities, subjects and budget) available to answer this question?

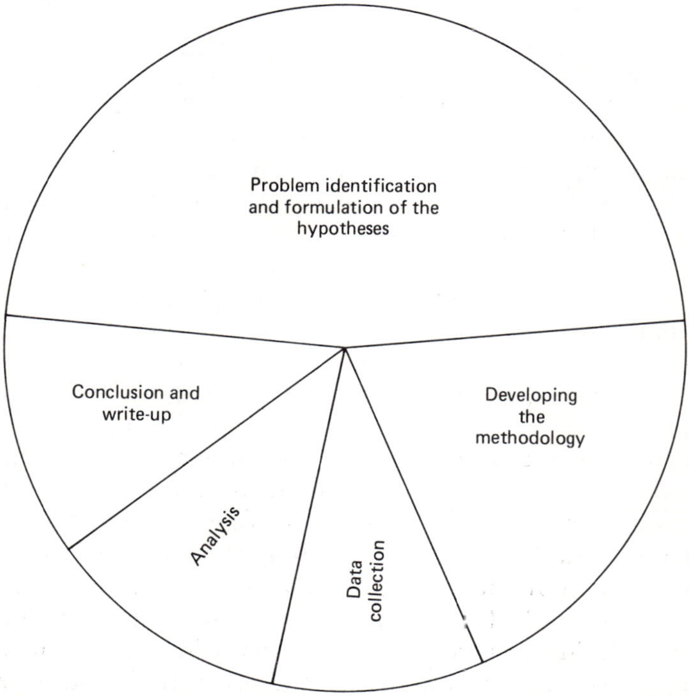

Figure 3-2. Proportion of time spent in the steps of the research process.

2. Is the support and cooperation of others (superiors, consultants, agencies, subjects) operative?
3. What difference will the answer to these questions make a) to patient care? b) To the education of health professionals? c) To further research?

In summary, a question well stated is a question half answered.

Once interesting, relevant, and specific questions are proposed, an investigator may speculate on the possible answers to the question. This speculative process of advancing propositions is the process of hypotheses generation. Many of the hypotheses which represent all the possible outcomes of a question can be answered by a careful review of the literature. Gaps in the literature will reveal hypotheses about a specific population of interest that have not been tested. A brief discussion of the review of literature and hypotheses development steps of research follows.

The Literature Review

Before beginning the library search it is helpful to plan a strategy for approaching the literature. The growth of knowledge in the past few years has been exponential (exponential value = the constant number raised to a given power). Thus, reviewing the literature with some focus provided by the specifically stated study question(s) is a useful approach. In any well stated question, an investigator identifies the "what?" to be investigated about "whom? where? when?" and "how?" The "why?" is pursued through a critique of the relevant literature.

An example of a question for study may be, "Is the health service utilization pattern (what) of frequent attenders (who) at family practices (where) during the course of a year (when) related to (how) those same persons' high level of emotional distress (what)?" A specifically stated question identifies the content or variable for investigation. This same content should be reviewed in the literature to elaborate the "why" of the investigation.

In the above example, the literature on health service utilization and emotional distress is abundant. In this case, the student may plan to define further these two broad fields by confining the review to the 1) population of interest (frequent attenders) and/or the 2) place of interest (family practice). This kind of "focusing" can result in three or four criteria or guidelines for approaching the literature. Adding the criterion "research of" or "outcome studies of" to a given content area is a fifth approach which is useful in further delineating the literature to be reviewed. Finally, if research in a given field is still abundant, the literature review may be confined to the last three or four years of publication or still further, by the type of research conducted.

For example, the literature on nurse practitioners has grown abundantly in the decade of the 1970s. While much of this literature is opinion based, even the research based literature is voluminous. A variety of approaches to research (descriptive, survey, and random controlled trials) were used in evaluating the patient outcomes of care by nurse practitioners. To deal with the problem of a variety of approaches, the review of the literature might include only those studies that employed the most rigorous design and methodology—the clinical trial (random assignment of subjects to experimental and control groups). The review would, therefore, exclude studies of nurse practitioners using other research designs (for example, surveys). Table 3-1 provides an example of how this literature and others might be summarized succinctly by size of sample, type of design, and variables investigated. The following discussion provides suggestions for critiquing the literature and identifying the hypotheses that have not been tested.

Table 3-1 indicates that both patient outcomes and professional activities were regularly emphasized as important variables in randomized controlled trials of nurse practitioners in ambulatory care. Invariably the studies have shown either no difference between nurses and physicians in patient outcomes or an improvement in the outcomes of patients receiving the care of the nurse. Nurse practitioner studies have not:

1. Been conducted with large samples
2. Provided thorough economic analyses of both direct and indirect costs and benefits of this pattern of health care from a variety of points of view (third party, the patient, society)
3. Tested the usefulness of community nurses functioning in this role
4. Tested community nurses' usefulness in managing the *frequent attender* patient population. These hypotheses would be tested in the proposed investigation.

As demonstrated in the foregoing example, one identifies from the literature what is known and not known about the area(s) of investigation. This analysis of the literature may lead to a refinement of the initial question(s). Chapter 5 discusses the literature review process more fully.

The literature critique generally addresses the quality of the design and method used in conducting the study, the type and size of the sample studies and the variables or content that were or were not investigated. This process of critiquing the literature is described more fully in Chapter 15. From the analysis of evidence in the literature on a given topic, speculation can be made about the outcome of the

Table 3-1. Summary of the Nurse Practitioner Random-Controlled Trials by Major Variables

	Type of Design	Professional Time Spent in All Activities		Patient Outcomes				
							Referral Patterns	
Number of Nurse Practitioners by Study	*Random-Control Trials*	*Nurses*	*All Professionals*	*Quality of Care: N.P. vs. M.D.*	*Health Status: N.P. vs. M.D.*	*Health Service Utiliza-tion: N.P. vs. M.D.*	*To Nsg*	*To M.D.*
Chambers, et al 1977 *N* = 6	X	X	X	O	O	O	X	X
Burnip, et al 1976 *N* = 6	X	X	X	O	O	O	////	////
Hockelman 1975 *N* = 3	X	X	X	O	O	O	////	////
Spitzer, et al 1975 *N* = 2	X	X	X	O	O	+	X	X

Schlesinger, et al 1973 $N = 3$	X	X	X	O	O	////	////	////
Yankauer, et al 1972 $N = 73$	X	X	////	O	////	////	////	////
Charney and Kitzman 1971 $N = 13$	X	X	X	O	O	O	////	////
Lewis, et al. 1969 $N = 2$	X	X	X	O	+	+	////	////

\+ = Patients assigned to the nurse show improved health status and reduced health service utilization compared with patients assigned to the physician.
O = No change in quality of care, health status, or health service utilization of patients assigned to the physician.
— = Patients assigned to the nurse worsened on some variable when compared with patients assigned to the physician.
//// = The variable was not tested.
X = The variable was measured or the type of study was conducted.

untested hypotheses. In this way hypotheses are advanced from the review of the literature.

FORMING HYPOTHESES

Explanations about how phenomena (variables) are related and/or affect each other are hypotheses. Hypotheses are statements of relationships among phenomena. Popper (1968) stated that whenever one proposes a relationship, one should attempt to propose either the opposite or alternative relationship rather than defend the relationship originally advanced.

A prediction of a relationship among variables in the form of an hypothesis can be stated as if it is to be "verified" by the study or "falsified" by the study. As Popper (1968) suggests, an hypothesis should be accompanied by the rival or alternate hypothesis to limit the bias of the investigator or a "chance result." The need for a rival or alternative hypothesis may arise. An example of this is given.

If it were hypothesized that all swans are white and, in sampling from the population of swans in one lake only white swans were discovered, then this proposition may be erroneously "verified" by "chance finding" or by "selection tendency" associated with the lake. In contrast, if the hypothesis stated that all swans are not white in an attempt to falsify the real conjecture or research hypotheses, then the methodology would provide for the selection of some nonwhite swans. This is a simple example of attempting to overthrow the solution rather than defend it or, in short, test the research hypotheses by gathering data on the alternative hypothesis (see the section on "Null Hypothesis" in Chap. 6).

Thus, as a first principle, the hypothesis must be stated in a form that can be tested versus verified. Further, an hypothesis must:

- Be stated in terms that are measurable
- Be free of value statements, for example, " . . . better than . . ."
- Specify the criteria that will either reject or accept the hypothesis, and
- Specify the two variables or the two groups being compared.

As an example, note the following conjecture and hypotheses which can be generated from a review of the literature on nurse practitioners for the foregoing criteria:

Research (H_R) hypothesis or general conjecture: the use of family practice and hospital services by frequent attenders is significantly reduced ($p < 0.05$) among those patients randomly assigned to receive the care of the nurse practitioner compared with those patients assigned to receive care from the physician.

Rival or alternative (H_A) hypotheses: the *reduction* in the amount of *health service utilization* among frequent attenders receiving care from nurse practitioners *compared with* those of patients receiving care from physicians is the same ($p > 0.05$).

The rival hypothesis is one advanced as the alternative hypothesis to the research hypothesis (reduced health service utilization). The variable is stated in measurable terms with the direction for the change clearly indicated. In this case, two groups of patients are being compared for differences. This example highlights the kind of statistical test to be conducted—a test of difference.

The criterion for accepting or rejecting an hypothesis is often a probability of 0.05 (5 in 100 chances) that such findings are due to chance alone. In other words, the hypothesis is either upheld, accepted, supported, or rejected. No value ladened words are used to describe the prediction or relationship. In any kind of hypothesis, only one comparison can be described at a time. If more comparisons are planned then additional hypotheses must be stated.

Once well-stated hypotheses are advanced, the plan for the type of data to be gathered becomes quite clear. Chapter 6 presents a full discussion of hypotheses development.

ORGANIZING AN APPROACH TO GATHERING THE DATA

Research methodology refers to the procedures and the sequence of procedures an investigator uses to conduct the study (gathering data on the variables outlined in the hypothesis or study question and analyzing the findings). The research methodology section of a report generally describes the:

- Setting of the study
- Design of the study (exploratory, correlational, experimental)
- Method of drawing a sample of patients from the larger population of interest
- Rationale for the size of the sample planned
- Time frame or calendar in which procedures are conducted
- Instrumentation used to measure the variables under scrutiny with some discussion of the assumptions underlying and the advantages and disadvantages of various measurement approaches or devices.

A study can stand or fall on the basis of the quality of the data which represent or tap the reality (variable) being tested. For example, an investigator can interview patients for the number of times they visited the doctor or actually count the number of times patients came to the doctor. Which source of data can be said to be more reliable? Given the inaccuracy of a patient's memory, a more reliable set of data would be an actual count of patient visits from the patient record. The beginning investigator is concerned not only with how to gather data from what source and when, but also with how to keep the rules about the manner in which these procedures are carried out with the subjects.

Subjects may be interviewed, or data may be gathered from patient records. Using records could be one way that minimizes bias. Conversely, an inexperienced investigator may carry out these data collection procedures in a way that is haphazard, not repeatable, or filled with errors. When the procedures are haphazard, a study is said to have extraneous variables operating that confound the findings. These extraneous variables are sources of error that:

- Negatively or positively affect the study subjects
- Conveniently approach only cooperative subjects
- Change the order of or timing of measuring subjects with instruments
- Gather data or rate subjects in two different ways.

The kinds of error produced by these factors involve breaking methodological rules and are referred to as sources of "invalidity (see Chap. 8)."

Validity in research can be classified as internal validity and external validity. Isaac and Michael (1978, p. 14) stated: "Internal Validity asks the question: did, in fact, the experimental treatment make a difference in this instance? External Validity asks the question: to what populations, settings, treatment variables, and measurement variables can this effect be generalized?"

Isaac and Michael have simplified Campbell and Stanley's (1973) classification of extraneous variables which produce invalidity in research results. These are summarized in Figure 3-3.

Not all of these sources of potential error can be controlled in all research. However, the more these sources of error are minimized by keeping the rules in the methodology, the more rigorous, conclusive, and generalized are the research results. For a more complete discussion of the types of research designs that minimize these sources of error, see Chapter 7. The validity of measurement devices (content validity, criterion validity, and construct validity) is discussed in detail in Chapters 8 and 9.

Once a procedure for gathering data has been completed, the next tasks include determining the size of the sample of subjects to measure and the procedures to analyze the data in a way that tests the hypotheses

INTERNAL VALIDITY

1. History—specific events occurring between the first and second measurement in addition to the experimental variable.
2. Maturation—processes within the subjects operating as a function of the passage of time, per se (growing older, hungrier, fatigued, or less attentive).
3. Testing—the effects of testing upon the scores of a subsequent testing.
4. Instrumentation—changes in obtained measurement due to changes in instrument calibration or changes in the observers or judges.
5. Statistical regression—a phenomenon occurring when groups have been selected on the basis of extreme scores.
6. Selection—biases resulting from the differential selection of subjects for the comparison groups.
7. Experimental mortality—the differential loss of subjects from the comparison groups.
8. Selection-maturation interaction, etc.—interaction effects between the aforementioned variables which can be mistaken for the effects of the experimental variable.

EXTERNAL VALIDITY

1. Interaction effects of selection biases and the experimental variable.
2. Reactive or interaction effect of pretesting—the pretesting modifies the subject in such a way that he responds to the experimental treatment differently than will unpretested persons in the same population.
3. Reactive effects of experimental procedures—effects arising from the experimental setting which will not occur in nonexperimental settings.
4. Multiple-treatment interference—effects due to multiple treatments applied to the same subjects where prior treatments influence subsequent treatments in the series because their effects are not erasable.

Figure 3-3. Sources of internal and external invalidity to be controlled in the research methodology. (Isaac, S., and Michael, W.B. *Handbook in Research and Evaluation.* San Diego: EdITS/Knapp Publisher, 1971. All rights reserved. Reproduced with permission.)

that were advanced. The following discussion elaborates some of the perspectives used when approaching these tasks.

Sample Size

There are a number of scientific approaches to determining sample size depending on the type of research design planned. Determining the sample for survey research differs from the procedures used in experimental or comparative research.

In survey research, sample size considerations are related to the degree of certainty with which the sample results represent the true population values of the variable in question. The *error rate* specifies how close we want the sample and population values to be. For example, an error rate of ±0.05 would mean that a sample result of 35% in favor of decreasing nurse time in the schools indicates a *true* value for the population of 30–40%. The *confidence level* specifies the probability that the sample results are not due to chance, but rather the results do reflect the true value within the error limits set. One can be 95% confident that results obtained are not due to chance.

By setting an estimated *expected* result for any one variable, plus the error rate and the confidence level, sample sizes can be calculated. It turns out that an expected 50/50 split on a yes or no question yields the largest sample size, and this is used here. The error rate is set at ±0.05 or ±0.10 and the confidence level at 95%.

The conceptual representation for Cockran's (1977) formula used to calculate sample size (n) in survey research is

Estimated sample for a survey design (n)

$$= \left(\frac{z \text{ value at 95\% confidence}}{5\% \text{ error rate}} \right)^2 \times \text{50–50 probability} \qquad \text{(II)}$$

Assigning numerical values for confidence, probability, and error in this case, the equation is:

$$n = (1.96/0.05)^2 \times (0.05)(0.05)$$

Solving this equation the estimated sample (n) equals:

$$n = 384$$

Where the size of the population (N) is small, correction can be made for finite population size. Cochran (1977) said that where N is not large, then:

$$n = \frac{n_0}{1 + (n_0 - 1)/N}$$

Other approaches to determining sample size in experimental research are elaborated in Chapter 9.

ANALYZING THE DATA

Popper (1968, p. 268) has stated that: "Analysis is . . . the appraisal of data . . . the statement about which either corroborates or falsifies hypotheses . . . We cannot define a numerical calculable degree of corroboration but we can speak only roughly in terms of positive . . . and negative degrees of corroboration."

Data can be analyzed in a number of ways. The crucial analyses are, however, those that test the hypotheses being advanced or the question asked. Consider the lack of logical analysis in the following example:

The research hypothesis states that patients in Group A and Group B experience the same level of health status ($p < 0.05$).

The criterion for judging difference or no difference is set at 0.05. If the probability of the finding is greater than 0.05 then the judgement of no difference, or "sameness," is made. To test this hypothesis the logical statistic should be one testing difference, yet the analysis reported is one of relationship between patients' health and use of services.

The result about relationships is interesting and noteworthy but it fails to test the issue of difference advanced in the hypothesis. A useful procedure to avoid this all too common pitfall is to restate the hypothesis and draw a "dummy table" (Table 3-2) to serve as a guide when summarizing and assembling data for presentation. The statistical test planned can be indicated beneath the table and in the case of the above example the statistical test should be one of "difference" versus "relationship." For example:

Hypothesis$_A$: patients in group A and group B experience the same level of health ($P < 0.05$).

Table 3-2. Health Status Differences Between Two Groups of Patients

Health Status	*Group A Patients*	*Group B Patients*	*Total*
Good			
Fair			
Poor			
Total			*N*

N = Total number of patients.
Test of difference = chi square χ^2
2 degrees of freedom.

This use of a dummy table as a planning device will expedite the analysis phase. The number of patients' scores indicating a "good" health status in Group A would be inserted in the appropriate box. This procedure continues until the boxes or "cells" are filled. Following Maxwell's (1975) formula for the computation of the chi square statistic testing "difference," a number is produced. The value of the chi square is found in a chi square table (see tables in the Appendix) and its value will show if the probability of obtaining this number is greater or less than alpha (α) or .05.

The criteria for rejecting the hypothesis of sameness at the α 0.05 (or if preferred α 0.01 level) are the numbers listed in these tables. If the research hypothesis of sameness is falsified or "rejected" by applying the numerical criteria from the table then the alternative hypothesis of difference between groups of patients is accepted or confirmed.

TYPE I AND TYPE II ERRORS

Concerning the hypothesis, there are two types of errors that the researcher may make. Type I error occurs when the researcher rejects an hypothesis that is actually true, and Type II error occurs when the investigator fails to reject a false hypothesis. The chance of making these types of error can be minimized by setting criteria for accepting or rejecting hypotheses within a designated region of distribution of scores of a population.

For example, consider the visual representation of two alternative sets of fictitious scores that could be made by a fictitious population (Fig. 3-4).

It is customary to set $\alpha = 0.05$ or 0.01. Then, if a given result falls in the area (5% or 1%) specified by α, the alternative hypothesis is rejected. If the hypothesis is true, a result falling in the region of rejection is possible but extremely unlikely. At $\alpha = 0.05$, 5% of the observed results will fall into the area of rejection by chance. Five out of every 100 true hypotheses will be rejected if we use the criterion of $\alpha = 0.05$. At $\alpha = 0.01$, the probability of this Type I error is once in every 100 tests. It would be wise to make α smaller but, unfortunately, there are also errors of the second kind, or Type II errors. A Type II error consists of failing to reject a false alternative hypothesis (Freeman, 1965). As with alpha, it is customary to set beta (β) at 0.10 or 0.20 to minimize the chance of making this error.

The probability that Type I and Type II errors will be made is inversely related. This can be interpreted to mean that when the risk of

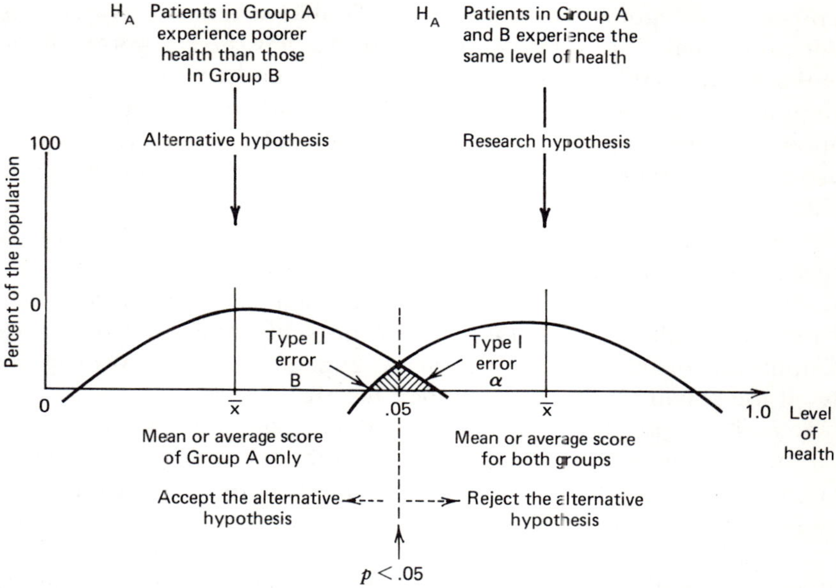

Figure 3-4. The distribution of scores for two populations.

making a Type I error is minimized, the chance of making a Type II error is greater. Treece and Treece (1977) stated that the probability of making a Type II error is also inversely related to sample size. When the sample size is increased, the researcher is able to reduce the probability of making a Type II error. See Chapter 6, Figure 6-1, and Part 3 of this book for clarification and an elaboration of these ideas.

STATISTICS

The question of which type of statistic to use when testing hypotheses is best answered by another question, what type of data are involved?

There are four types of data:

1. Nominal data
2. Ordinal data
3. Interval data
4. Ratio data

Nominal data can be called descriptive or categorical data, according to Kerlinger (1973). Observations about variables are classified into the appropriate category. For example, the variable, sex, has two categories, male and female; the variable, marital status, has the categories single, common-law, married, separated, divorced, and widowed. In each example, the categories are 1) mutually exclusive (meaning an observation can be classified in only one category) and 2) collectively exhaustive (meaning there are sufficient categories to accommodate every possible observation).

Ordinal data not only describes a variable in categories but also an arrangement of categories in degrees of occurence of a variable. For example, there cannot be degrees of a marital state but there can be degrees of health, satisfaction, or adequacy of clinical performance. Examples of ordinal scales are 1) least, 2) somewhat, and 3) most like myself, or 1) bad, 2) fair, and 3) good health.

Interval data extend beyond ordinal data. Interval data are ordered and the difference between each point on the scale is known and equal. This is not true of the ordinal scale. Some examples of the interval scale are the thermometer, the specific gravity measurement scale, age expressed in years, weight, milligrams of glucose in the blood, etc. The student can easily understand the nature of this scale by considering ages: a person could be 1 year and 6 months or 1 year and 7 months.

Finally, ratio data and the ratio scale have all the properties of the previous scales and, in addition, have the property of an absolute zero point. Referring to the examples of interval scale above, there can be no natural or true zero units of age or weight. The zero may apply, however, to money, for example, expenses or costs, where there is a true zero point. For further discussion of these four scales, see the section in Chapter 10 on "Instruments For Data Collection."

Specifying the type of data to be collected is important because only certain nonparametric statistics should be used with nominal data. Kerlinger (1973) extends this rule to include ordinal data, while both nonparametric and parametric statistics can be used with interval and ratio data. Some statisticians believe that determining scales is secondary to plotting the data. However, beginning investigators usually rely on the type of scale that their data fit.

Figure 3-5 outlines a simple way to remember the type of statistic that is applicable to the type of data or measurement scale.

As shown in Figure 3-5, to test hypotheses of relationships between variables, either the Spearman Rank Order Correlation or the Pearson Product Moment Correlation is appropriate to use, depending on the *type* of data being tested (Lathrop, 1969). The topic of statistics (parametric and nonparametric) is elaborated in Chapters 12 and 13.

Type of Data or Scale	*Type of Statistics*	*Examples*	*Symbol*	*Meaning of Each Statistic*
Nominal	Nonparametric	Frequencies	f	The *amount*, percent, or proportion of an observation
		Percentages	%	
		Proportion	p_2	
		chi square	x	The *difference* between observations
Ordinal	/////	Pearson rank-order correlation	r_s	The *relationship* between variables
Interval	Parametric	t-test	t	The *difference* between two means
Ratio		F-Ratio	F	The *variance* among or between populations on a given variable
		Pearson product moment correlation	r	The *relationship* between variables

///// = area of disagreement among statisticians

Figure 3-5. The relationship between the type of research data and the type of statistics that is appropriate.

SUMMARY

This chapter has introduced the beginning investigator to the basic approaches to scientific inquiry. This presentation has centered on the types of research, the problem for study and the specific literature to be reviewed, hypothesis writing, methodological rules to insure valid and reliable results, and the use of dummy tables as a guide in analyzing results. In the remainder of this book, the student will find a more detailed discussion of each step of the research process introduced here. These steps provide an outline of the research process.

BIBLIOGRAPHY

Bacon, F. *Novum Organum,* Book 1. Chicago: Great Books Foundation, Henry Regnery Company, 1949.

Best, J. W., *Research in Education* (2nd Ed.). New Jersey: Prentice-Hall, Inc., 1970.

Burnip, R., Erickson, R. & Barr, G.D. Well-child care by pediatric nurse practitioners in a large group practice. *American Journal of Diseases of Children,* January, 1976, *130.* Pp. 51-55.

Campbell, D., & Stanley, J. *Experimental and Quasi-Experimental Designs for Research.* Chicago: Rand-McNally Publishing Co., 1966.

Chambers, L. W., & West, A.E. *The St. John's Randomized Trial of the Family Practice Nurse: Methodological Manual and Final Report.* Unpublished monograph, McMaster University, August, 1977.

Charney, E., & Kitzman, H. The child-health nurse (pediatric nurse practitioner) in private practice: a controlled trial. *New England Journal of Medicine,* 1971, *285,* Pp. 1353-1358.

Cockran, W. G. *Sampling Techniques* (3rd Ed.). Toronto: John Wiley & Sons, 1977. Pp. 74-77.

Freeman, L. C. *Elementary Applied Statistics for Students in the Behavioural Sciences.* New York: John Wiley & Sons, 1965. Pp. 154-156.

French, R. M. *The Dynamics of Health Care.* New York: McGraw-Hill Book Company, 1968. Pp. 112.

Gathrop, R. C. *Introduction to Psychological Research.* New York: Harper and Row Publishers, 1969. Pp. 1-27.

Hoekelman, R. A. What constitutes adequate well-baby care? *Pediatrics,* March, 1975, *55*(3), pp. 313-326.

Isaac, S. & M. W. *Handbook in Research and Evaluation.* San Diego: Edits Publishers, 1978. Pp. 14.

Kerlinger, F. N. *Foundations of Behavioural Research* (2nd ed.). Toronto: Holt, Rinehart and Winston, 1973. Pp. 39-40, 435-439.

Lathrop, R. E. *Introduction to Psychological Research.* New York: Harper and Row, 1969. Pp. 200-219.

Lewis, C. E., Resnik, B.A., & Schmidt, G. Activities, events and outcomes in ambulatory patient care. *The New England Journal of Medicine,* March 20, 1969, *280*(12), pp. 645-649.

Maxwell, A. E. *Analyzing Qualitative Data.* London: Chapman and Hall, Science Paper Backs, 1975. Chapter 1.

Organ, T. W. *The Art of Clinical Thinking.* Boston: Houghton Mifflin Company, 1965. Pp. 199-207.

Popham, W. J. *Evaluation in Education.* Berkeley: McCutchan Publishing Corporation, 1974.

Popper, K. R. *The Logic of Scientific Discovery* (2nd ed.). New York: Harper and Row Publishers, 1968. Pp. 16, 268.

Schatzman, L., & Strauss, A. *Field Research.* New Jersey: Prentice-Hall, Inc., 1973.

Schlesinger, E. R., Lowers, W.D. & Glaser, D.B. A controlled test of the use of registered nurses for prenatal care. *Health Services Reports,* May, 1973, *88*(5), pp. 400-404.

Spitzer, W. O., Sackett, D. L., Sibley, J. C., Roberts, R. S., Gent, M., Kergin, D. J., Hackett, B. C., & Olynich, A. The Burlington randomized trial of the nurse practitioner. *New England Journal of Medicine,* 1975, *290,* pp. 251-256.

Treece, E. W., & Treece, J. W. *Elements of Research in Nursing.* St. Louis: The C. V. Mosby Company, 1973. P. 5; 1977. Pp. 261-262.

Whitehead, A. N. *Adventures of Ideas.* New York: The Free Press, 1967. Pp. 140-159.

Yankauer, A., Tripp, S., Andrews, J.P. The outcomes and service impact of a pediatric nurse practitioner training program—nurse practitioner training outcomes. *American Journal of Public Health,* March, 1972, *62,* pp. 347-353.

4
Theories, Concepts, and Nursing Practice

Knowledge about the role of theory in the advancement of science is essential for the development of a profession and for the conduct of research. This is true for the nursing profession as well as for other professions. Recently nursing has reported its research on theory development in the literature and through nursing conferences. Journals such as *Nursing Research* and *Research in Nursing and Health* have provided sources for publication on the development of theories. Also, in recent years there has been a proliferation of conferences on nursing theory. These conferences focus heavily on nursing theory and the clinical research necessary for its advancement. This concern with nursing theory began in the mid-1960s, received a substantial boost in 1968 from Dickhoff, James, and Wiedenback, and in 1970 from Rogers, and has been gathering momentum ever since. Along with such conferences, the Western Interstate Commission on Higher Education (WICHE), of which nursing is a branch (WICHEN), has contributed to this momentum.

Thus far, most of the work on theory development has been related to nursing care and nursing education. In an applied discipline like nursing, emphasis must be placed on the preparation of professionals and on practice; therefore, the discipline dictates that investigation in nursing theory not only be related to patient status and care but also to nursing education and nursing performance. Presumably, the student needs to know and be encouraged to accept the broad areas of research. Continued interest and effort in theory development is needed and will result in the further advancement of nursing knowledge and expertise. The purpose of this chapter is to present an overview of theory and its relationship to nursing research and practice. The chapter begins with a discussion of theories, especially those used in nursing practice, followed by a discussion of concepts and their role in research. Finally, a problem in public health nursing practice is given to illustrate the application of the general systems theory.

THEORIES

An Overview

Webster defines a theory as "a formulation of apparent relationships or underlying principles of certain observed phenomena which has been verified to some degree." Theories should be the foundation on which research is developed. Theories become comprehensive and explicit through ongoing research. Therefore, there is a *seesaw* effect of theory development and valid investigation. Theories may have a personal, historical, sociologic (cultural), or philosophic basis (French, 1974). Their function is to organize and explain the relationship of questions whose answers (when validated) lead to new knowledge. Theories guide people's observations about the world.

The importance of guiding people's observations about the world can be illustrated by the following examples. Consider the effects of Pasteur's germ theory and Darwin's theory of generation. Pasteur's work formed the basis for considering the causes, containment, and prevention of disease. Darwin's theory of evolution helped to develop the agent, host, and environment method for investigating the distribution of diseases. These theories have been important to the science of epidemiology. Other theories that have become important to science are the Newtonian theory in physics and Einstein's theory of relativity. In considering these theories and many others, it can be seen that theories "enable predictions to be tested and choices to be made between paths of actions," and thus they advance science and guide the conduct of research (Susser, 1973, p. 13). Therefore, it is important to understand how theories may be developed.

There are two approaches or strategies for developing theory: inductive and deductive (see Chap. 3). The inductive approach involves developing the research and then the theory. In essence it includes answering a question or questions and then explaining the relationships revealed by theoretical formulation. The second strategy is to develop the theory and then conduct research to substantiate or disprove the theory. This is the deductive approach (Susser, 1973). This chapter will consider only the first of these two approaches.

Developing theory as a result of research efforts requires that the investigator proceed through the following steps: 1) select a phenomenon or problem and identify its characteristics, 2) measure the characteristics in a variety of settings, 3) analyze the data to ascertain patterns that are systematic and therefore warrant further attention, and 4) when patterns are found, formalize them into axioms (basic statements) (Reynolds, 1971). Basic statements that are derived from axioms are called propositions.

One type of theory that is often used in nursing is systems theory, which may be described as a theory that focuses on a set or group of components or processes that are interactive and closely related. This may be likened to an outline in which a main topic is supported by related sections. In systems theory the related sections of the outline are called the subsystems. The theory presupposes that the relationships or interactions of the subsystems explain, contribute to, or cause outcomes (the main topic) of an outline. However, unlike an outline, systems theory has final results that can be considered equal. In other words, if all else is equal, then all outcomes of the subsystems are equal too. This can be understood using an example of an objective and subobjectives related to a health problem. Consider the achievement of the broad objective, "to improve the vision of patients attending an eye clinic." To meet that objective, the nurse considers several subobjectives. These may include the arrangement of more convenient clinic hours, transportation, and affordable glasses for those who need financial assistance. Each subobjective alone would meet a part of the objective. Quantification of the outcome would be in terms of effort (the development of subobjectives), and success would be in terms of achieving the major objective. Each subobjective would have an equal impact on the final success of meeting the overall objective. Another way of viewing or expressing it would be that any one of a set of alternatives has equal probability of achieving the objective. This is the principle of equifinality, and it is a critical proposition of systems theory. It is relevant to various study designs and is frequently used as the basic proposition of investigation.

Early work using systems theory was conducted by Bales and Homans. Bales developed an observational scheme to study the interaction process among small groups. He suggested that group members who communicate accomplish their tasks and build solidarity as opposed to those who do not (Shepherd, 1964). Homans began his theory development with the study of the concepts of interaction, activity, and sentiments. He then investigated the interaction among people in small groups, using those concepts as a beginning point of investigation (Homans, 1950). Bales and Homans tested their concepts by observing and recording the interaction among group members. With sufficient testing to indicate that the concepts were valid, the researchers were able to conclude that they had developed a theory of interaction among small groups. In addition to Bales and Homans, other investigators have developed theories related to systems of interaction among small groups. The reader is urged to refer to texts of social psychology, such as that written by Hollander and Hunt, for additional information about small group theories.

The assumptive base allows an investigator to decide the focus of interest. The dictates of nursing process coincide with the assumptions of systems theory. Students should identify the assumptions that dictate goal setting, planning, implementing, and evaluating the nursing process.

Theories in Nursing

An overview of theory was introduced in the preceding section, indicating theory development. This section presents a discussion of theories that may be used in nursing.

General systems theory is a theory of action. The action can be determined by investigating the input, output, and evaluation of the system under study. One must consider the effects of the subsystems in the input, output, and evaluation of the action, always providing for feedback so that action can be adjusted when necessary (Fuerst, et al, 1974). General systems theory applied to nursing provides some assistance in determining the type of care to be given to patients. It is based on patient care goals and the methods used to reach them. The process used to attain the goals of patient care in relation to systems theory can be stated as follows:

1. *Set immediate goals,* considering dangers to the patient and establishing patient priorities. This step may involve only the nurse, if the patient is too ill to participate.
2. *Plan* nursing strategy based on the goals.
3. *Implement* patient care by those most qualified to provide it. This could include other nurses, family members, or the patients themselves.
4. *Evaluate* the outcome of the patient care in terms of the goals set. Were the goals attained or, if not, to what extent? If not, the nurse asks why not? Were the goals realistic? Was the planning unrealistic? Was the research attitudinal, evaluative? Was implementation inadequate? If the goals were attained, the nursing process either ends or proceeds to more ambitious goals (Vailott, 1970).

The assumptive base of systems theory allows an investigator to decide the focus of interest. The dictates of the nursing process coincide with the assumptions of systems theory. Students should identify the assumptions that dictate goal setting and planning, implementing, and evaluating the nursing process.

General systems theory may provide the organization of direction or guidance for care given, if the system goals that are selected are patient centered. The identification of explicit objectives is critical to the usefulness of the theory. This is especially true for an investigator whose research objective is the observation and analysis of the nursing process, that is, the nursing actions, whether it is nursing-focused action or small-group interaction. General systems theory and nursing process are similar in their organizing approaches or frameworks. They explain or dictate very little of the content of the process or action. It is quite possible, however, for the clinician, as well as the investigator, to operate from the assumptive base of systems theory. For further examples of nursing theorists whose conceptual frameworks assume the systems base, the student is encouraged to consult King (1971) and Byrne and Thompson (1972). Another well established text by Yura and Walsh (1973) addresses the relationship of systems theory, nursing process, and interpersonal interaction. The nurses providing care in hospital and other settings may use tbe general systems theory as a framework for delivering nursing care.

Another theory or conceptual framework used in nursing practice is the self-care theoretical framework developed by Orem. This theoretical framework is based on the belief that "nursing has as its special concern man's need for self-care action and the provision and management of it on a continuous basis in order to sustain life and health, recover from disease or injury, and cope with their effects" (Orem, 1971, pp. 1–2). Self-care, so conceived, includes those activities that patients perform or can learn for themselves to enhance their health status.

In using the self-care theory as a basis for practice in a public health setting, the nurse would 1) assess the self-care status of the patient, 2) identify the objectives whose achievement would yield patient independence, 3) design a system of nursing care that contributes to the patient's achievement of self-care, and 4) organize and implement the necessary support strategies that would guarantee the patient's participation in enhancing his or her self-care capabilities. In other words, the nurse helps the patient move from his or her current situation to meet the health goals.

The nurse provides a diagnosis of the patient's interest in his or her own health care (Nos. 1 and 2) as well as his or her future ability to perform self-care activities (Nos. 3 and 4). The nursing process can be defined as those physical and mental activities in which the nurse engages for delivering patient care. The framework of the self-care theory consists of assisting, monitoring, adjusting, and evaluating the patient's activities in helping the patient to meet his or her health goals. It is a theory that depends on other theories that are related to the internal and external controls in the behaviors of people.

An additional nursing theoretical framework is based on an adaptation model developed by Roy. She views humankind as biopsychosocial beings who are in constant interaction with a changing environment. The model focuses on nursing's ability to assist people in their adaptation to their 1) changing physiologic needs, 2) self-concept, 3) role function, and 4) interdependence. Major elements of this model are the recipient of nursing care, the goal of nursing, and the activities that are needed to reach the nursing goal. The nursing activities include assessing patient behavior and factors that influence adaptation level and intervening when necessary (Roy, 1976).

Many of the current models for nursing practice have been presented in terms of the *criteria for an effective model.* These criteria were initially formulated, or organized, by Dickhoff and James (1970) and were presented in nursing terms by Johnson (1974). The recipient of nursing care is the patient; the nursing goal is to promote adaptation in the four modes listed above.

Additional theories of interest to the nurse may include those of Glaser and Strauss (1970), grounded theorists, as well as Rogers (1970) and Peplau (1952), nursing theorists. Each theory has a specific purpose applicable to nursing. It is suggested that the reader consult Verhonick (1975) for further discussion of nursing theories and their construction as a basis for research. Also, the reader may refer to Riehl (1974) and Roy (1976) for conceptual models.

CONCEPTS

Concepts play an essential role in the understanding of theories as well as in developing research. They are the building blocks of theory. For that role to be appreciated, concepts must be defined. A concept is an idea or thought that labels an abstract notion (see Chap. 6). The reader is urged to refer to Woodruff (1961) for further discussion.

Nursing process involves the need for many defined concepts. Let us consider a hypothetical example of this from nursing practice in a hospital. Patients are hospitalized for a surgical procedure. The notion of patients' fears about expected surgery may be interpreted differently by each patient. When two patients discuss those fears, it is likely that they will differ on the meanings. When asked, "How do you know when you are afraid?", one patient may respond, "My body shakes, my heart races, and I stutter over words." The other patient may describe it by saying, "I lose my appetite, I cry, I feel apprehensive, and I become suspicious." The nurses may interpret each patient's response as an inability to think and act appropriately. It can be seen that the idea of being afraid is expressed differently in each instance, depending on the person and the situation. However, there is a similarity in the responses that leads one to think they may be describing the same phenomenon—fear. It is suggested that fear is a concept. This is a useful mental abstract that permits the clinician to identify patient behavior from a pattern of attributes. Also, it allows the researcher to describe variables for study and gives the theorist a formulation to consider in relation to other phenomena.

In this example, the idea of fear is defined individually and those definitions are based on the person's perceptions, feelings, and responses. It can be said that fear as a concept is an abstraction of ideas that gives meaning to perceptions, feelings, and responses. It began as a word (fear) and would be stored in the memory bank for future use (King, 1971). Perceptions, feelings, and responses help to formulate concepts. They are the "process by which senses transmit meaning to the brain" (King, 1971, p. 12).

The preceding discussion briefly presents the foundation for concept development. However, defining the word *concept* may be problematic. The Random House Dictionary defines it as "a general notion or idea" and "an idea of something formed by mentally obtaining all of its characteristics or particulars." Webster's states that a concept is "an idea or thought, especially a generalized idea of a class of objects; abstract notion." In defining concepts, one can look to the dictionaries for "real" definitions. These definitions depict the essence of the meaning or the "real characteristics of the object or phenomenon" (Reynolds, 1971, p. 48). The assumption is that the object has real properties that can be described. The racing heart, crying, and apprehension were real characteristics of fear in the example cited earlier, and they can be used to describe fear. Another example would be nursing. This concept can be mentally pictured by such properties as giving a bath, making the person comfortable, and teaching about diet (Ford, Cobb, and Taylor,

1967). These are real properties, which can be identified and measured. Thus, it can be said that a concept is a representation of reality. Concepts seem difficult, but they are essential to communication.

Concepts may be communicated in many ways, such as through body language, speaking, and writing. In nursing, communication is often accomplished through writing (research, patients' health records, etc.). Communicating a concept in writing requires that it be observable or measurable. If a concept is defined as an abstraction of all the characteristics an object has in common, then the characteristics must be observable or measurable. It is essential to specify the particulars about the abstraction so that others will understand what is meant. For example, the concept of chair is easy to define; the concept of nurse is more difficult. It can be said that the greater the distance between concepts and the real world to which they refer, the greater the difficulty in developing or understanding their description. For example, to a skiing Northerner, there may be twelve kinds of snow; to a Southerner there is one kind. The concept of snow may be misunderstood and perhaps carelessly used by the Southerner.

An example of the difficulty of concept description can be illustrated with a frequently used, highly abstract concept: *man is becoming*. Man is becoming what? More attractive? Students may more clearly understand *becoming* if they would associate it with self-actualization. Faculty tend to refer to students' self-actualization in the same vein as students' *becoming*. The two concepts may be used interchangeably. Another abstract concept is *students will reach their maximum potential*. Maximum potential for what? Income? Honor grades? Concepts are needed to give general meaning to ideas, relate one fact to another, and relate findings to other studies having similar concepts. This is why they are important in research. Definitions are the boundaries of concepts. To be used in research, concepts need clear definitions so that data collected in a study are standardized, observable, and measurable. This can be achieved by making the definitions operational.

In research the function of operational definitions is to spell out and indicate the procedures used in measurement. They are indicators of the concept. "Nursing is what nurses do" is a poor definition and could not be called operational. It is circular, it fails to provide insight into the concept of nursing, and it is difficult to measure. Another poor operational definition is one that is manipulative. An example of this type can be shown by the hypothesis: Frustration leads to aggression. A manipulative definition of aggression would be that "it is the behavior that follows frustration." The reader learns nothing about the definition of either frustration or aggression. Attention to the development of clear operational definitions of concepts is essential for their understanding and use. An example of a good operational definition would be the following: "A *registered nurse* is one who has successfully passed a state examination for registered nurse licensure and is currently registered in the appropriate state." This definition is clear and measurable. Concepts lead to the development of hypotheses (see Chap. 6) for a proposed research project and to their fruitful comparison with findings from other studies. Poor definitions of concepts lead to false reports or at least increase the risk of misinterpretation.

The reader may see from the preceding examples that an array of concepts do not constitute a theory, but they "may enter a theoretic system" (Merton, p. 143). When concepts are interrelated in a scheme, the theory begins to emerge as the explication of the relationship. Nurses, along with other professional groups who are involved with research, must be aware of the role of concepts and their analyses in their research plan.

NURSING PRACTICE

Background

Nurses have a long heritage of caring for the ill. People have always been troubled with sickness of many kinds and have needed care, usually provided by well people. In early times, servants were hired not only to perform general tasks (farming, cooking, etc.) for their employers, but also to care for the sick members in the families. Eventually members of religious sects took over this function, and they invoked the spiritual and magical needs of the ill based on their religious and cultural traditions. Religious groups were followed by the military in providing care for the injured during major wars (Mausch, 1972).

The onset of modern nursing care based on knowledge began in the nineteenth century with the work of Florence Nightingale (1820–1910) in the Crimean War. It was during that war that Nightingale organized and gave care to injured English army soldiers, maltreated patients in the infirmaries, and the sick at home. Nightingale observed that her organizational efforts went hand in hand with the medical care given to these patients.

One century before the Crimean War there had been a humanitarian movement in England. In this movement, society focused its attention on certain underprivileged groups and attempted to improve their conditions. The publication of a document describing the sufferings of people from poverty, sickness, and child labor abuse was one result of this movement. The humanitarian movement, the Crimean War effort, and the belief that women should focus their attention on the bedside care of the sick and injured led Nightingale to feel that medical and social problems could be improved through the encouragement of women to become nurses (Sellew and Nuesse, 1951).

Nightingale described the care that she provided to patients during the Crimean War. In giving that care she noted the importance of the environment, including the cleanliness of the air, bed, and walls, as well as the noise and lighting in the rooms. Nightingale stressed, in addition to the environmental factors, the importance of observation of the sick for such things as diets, weakness states, and progression toward wellness. These observations were used to help save patients' lives, improve their health, and provide for their comfort. Nightingale firmly believed that the ability to observe was essential for nurses (Nightingale, 1970). Her major contributions to the care of the sick were advocating formal education for gaining the necessary knowledge to pursue a career in nursing and focusing on the patient rather than on the disease. The foundations for the profession of nursing had been laid.

Current Nursing Practice

Since Nightingale's initial work, the nursing profession has grown and changed a great deal. Nurses today still continue to use the caring and observation skills that Nightingale stressed; however, now they are formally educated for this role.

Preparation may be gained in a variety of formal educational programs that prepare nurses for various levels of knowledge and ability. These programs may be found in hospitals awarding diplomas, in community colleges awarding associate of arts degrees, or in universities or colleges conferring baccalaureate degrees. Advanced nursing education may include master's and doctoral degrees. Regardless of the type of educational setting, all graduates of nursing programs must sit for and pass a licensing examination in order to practice as registered nurses.

After registration, some nurses seek further education in specialty areas, such as pediatrics and midwifery, and some nurses have sought certification in these areas. Although nurses have expanded their nursing interests and intellectual competencies, they generally rely on Nightingale's original commitment to nursing care goals.

Nurses in practice today provide patient care in hospitals, public health agencies, nursing homes, industries, schools, Health Maintenance Organizations, or in the patients' homes. Each of these settings has a different organizational system, and most reimburse nurses through that system. One exception might be for nurses providing private care, in which the patient directly reimburses the nurse. However, in most of these settings it can hardly be said that nurses reap financial profit from their profession; thus the energy source for nursing activity must be more internal than external. It can be said that nurses rely on "internal forces" to provide patient or family care (Dickhoff and James, 1970). That care must be safe and satisfactory for patients, nurses, and organizations. The nurses' function is to assist patients through their infirmities, diseases, or dysfunctions (Schlotfeldt, 1971). One way to achieve these goals is through attentive application of the nursing process. In most of these settings nurses use the nursing process to deliver patient or family care.

The Nursing Process

Nursing care can be provided by a variety of nurses to patients in a variety of health care settings. The method by which that care is given is called the nursing process. The nursing process is defined as those physical and mental activities that the nurse employs to deliver patient or family care. It may also be defined as the "sum total of nursing care activities performed to aid in promoting the patient's well-being" (Fuerst, et al, 1974, p. 49). Nursing also takes place in the public health setting where the nursing process is based on systems theory.

The nursing process in the public health setting, as in any setting, should be provided in an organized and systematic manner. That process is based on the general systems theory described earlier in this chapter. The practicing or student Public Health Nurse (PHN) using this theory can begin by obtaining some facts about the community in which the family lives as well as the health agency for which the nurse works. These facts become the basis from which the nurse and patient or family can build health care goals. The community facts would include demographic information such as the community's geographic location in relation to the nearest large city, its water and sewage treatment facilities, its poverty level, its death and birth rates, the presence of chronic and infectious diseases, and resources. Resources would include public transportation, schools, police and fire departments, types of health agencies, and active community groups such as churches, Junior Chamber of Commerce, and so on. In addition to knowledge about the community, the PHN would need facts about the health agency in which she is employed, especially its services. This information would include types of services offered; types of patients distributed by age, sex, race, place of residence; and major health problems of the population receiving care. Once the PHN was well grounded in the pertinent community and agency facts, she would proceed with the nursing care of families.

In order to establish health care priorities for the families in his or her care, a PHN needs information that will become the basis for setting the immediate nursing care goals (an aspect of step 1 of the systems theory). This information may include 1) age and sex of the patient, 2) reasons for seeking health care, and 3) personal information about the family, such as its composition and its health history. The nurse would obtain a great deal of this information during the first interaction with the family.

Initial patient–PHN encounters usually occur in a specific clinic. However, they may occur in a family's home. Nurses often are assigned families to receive their care based on the geographic location of the families. The nurses already possess the community facts they need to provide effective care for their families. The nursing process that may be used in a community setting could assume the following pattern.

Suppose a patient is newly admitted to health care with suspected active tuberculosis (Tbc). The patient had noticed persistant chest pain and coughing. He is a 65-year-old childless married man with 12 years of education, and he is a farmer who has lived in a rural area all his life. When he becomes worried about his symptoms, he and his wife decide to visit the health department for a checkup. At that time he is seen by a PHN and a physician. A health history, physical examination, and chest x-ray are obtained. The suspicion of active tuberculosis is confirmed. The physician places the patient and his wife on medication. In this example the patient was self-referred, and his record began at the time of his initial visit. He was added to the PHN's caseload based on his place of residence.

The nurse sets immediate goals (phase 1 of systems theory) for the family to follow the doctor's recommendations. These recommendations would include the family maintaining the proper nutritional status and complying with the drug regimen. Also, the nurse sets goals based on the family's concern in living with and learning about tuberculosis. With the immediate goals set, the nurse advises the family that she will be making periodic home visits.

With the patient's chart reviewed and the immediate goals established, the PHN makes arrangements for a first home visit. This home visit provides time for the nurse to become more acquainted with the family and to assess their need for education about the disease. Also, the PHN gathers further background information on the patient, such as his home living conditions, cooking arrangements, work capability, recent contacts, and social activities. The nurse explains the importance of the patient's complying with his drug regimen as well as the safe care of contaminated materials. The nurse takes this opportunity to listen to the family's concern about tuberculosis, to answer their questions, and to assess the family needs. The nurse is able to plan strategies (phase 2 of the applied systems theory) for reaching the family goals.

During the course of the home visit, the nurse not only becomes acquainted with the family but also learns about their worries related to the patient's condition. These worries center on the husband's condition growing worse and his possible inability to continue working, the wife's insecurity about her knowledge related to preparing nutritious diets, and the handling of contaminated materials. Jointly, they are concerned about the past and future contamination of other people. With this additional information added to the patient's and family's data base, the PHN concludes that the family seems in need of 1) education about tuberculosis that would focus on nutrition and methods to avoid transmission of the disease, and 2) someone to help them discuss their fears about the effect of tuberculosis on the family, including the contamination of others and the loss of financial security. The PHN now can implement the nursing care (phase 3 of the systems theory) of this family.

To provide the identified needs for education related to the disease and to nutrition, as well as to be a supportive listener to discuss the family's fears, the nurse may intervene individually or call upon other health team members for assistance. In the event of need for other health team members, the nurse may ask for the assistance of a nutritionist, a psychiatric nurse, and a social worker. With or without the aid of other health care team members, the PHN provides education for the family regarding the importance of medication, the method by which the disease organism is transmitted, the level of isolation required to ensure the safety of others, and the prophylactic treatment of individuals who have been in contact with the patient. Clearly, the nurse provides surveillance of the family regarding compliance with prescribed medication (Freeman, 1970).

Overall, it can be said that the nursing care for this family can be defined by the nurse's actions taken as a result of her contact with the family. These actions would include fulfilling the family's educational needs about the disease and providing attentive listening as the family expresses concerns. The nurse would direct the family to other health care providers when needed. Further, the nurse would keep the family's health record in which the actions taken on the family's behalf would be described.

The health record provides a source for other workers to become knowledgeable about the current health status of the family. The nurse could feel reasonably secure that the family received care that was understood, appropriate, and coordinated. A basis for the evaluation (phase 4 of systems theory) of nursing care is established, and the nurse is now able to measure the effects of the care that was given to the family.

Using general systems theory in public health nursing has been dependent upon identifying immediate family health care goals, negotiating a compromise such as planning strategies, implementing tasks to achieve those goals, and evaluating the success of the process. The nursing care has been systematic, organized, and based on community and family data pertinent to the family health needs.

SUMMARY

In this chapter an overview of theories has been presented and their importance for advancing knowledge and a process for their development has been stressed. Selected theories developed by nurses were discussed. In addition, the role of concepts in theory development was presented. Finally, an example based on public health nursing care was given, illustrating the role of general systems theory in nursing practice. It has been shown that theories provide a foundation for nursing practice and research by helping nurses to build a sound scientific approach to the practice of various aspects of nursing.

BIBLIOGRAPHY

Byrne, M. L., & Thompson, L. F. *Key Concepts for the Study and Practice of Nursing.* St. Louis. The C. V. Mosby Co., 1972.

Dickhoff, J., James, P., & Wiedenbach, E. Theory in a practice discipline, Part I, Practice oriented theory, *Nursing Research,* September/October, 1968, *17,* pp. 62–92.

Dickhoff, J., & James, P. Beliefs and values: Bases for curriculum design. *Nursing Research,* September/October, 1970, *19,* No. 5, pp. 415–426.

Ford, L. C., Cobb, M., & Taylor, M. *Defining Clinical Content.* Boulder, Colorado: W.I.C.H.E., Feb., 1967.

Freeman, R. B. *Community Health Nursing Practice.* Philadelphia: W. B. Saunders Co., 1970.

French. R. M. *The Dynamics of Health Care,* 2nd Edition. New York: McGraw-Hill Book Co., 1974.

Fuerst, E. V., Wolff, L. V., & Weitzel, M. H. *Fundamentals of Nursing,* 5th Edition. Philadelphia: J. B. Lippincott Co., 1974.

Glaser, G. B., and Strauss, A. L. *The Discovery of Grounded Theory: Strategies for Qualitative Research.* 3rd Edition. Chicago: Aldine Publishing Co., 1970.

Hollander, E. P., & Hunt, R. G. (eds.), *Current Perspectives in Social Psychology,* 3rd Edition. New York: Oxford University Press, 1971.

Homans, G. C. *The Human Group.* New York: Harcourt, Brace & World, Inc., 1950.

Johnson, D., Development of theory: A requisite for nursing as a primary health profession. *Nursing Research,* September/October, 1974, *23,* pp. 372–377.

King, I. M. *Toward a Theory for Nursing.* New York: John Wiley & Sons, 1971.

Mausch, O. Nursing: Churning for Change? in Freeman, H. E., Levine, S., & Reeder, L. G., (eds.), *Handbook of Medical Sociology,* 2nd Edition. Englewood Cliffs, New Jersey: Prentice-Hall, Inc., 1972.

Merton, R. K. *Social Theory & Social Structure.* New York: The Free Press, 1968.

Nightingale, F. *Notes on Nursing.* London: Brandon/Systems Press, Inc., 1970.

Orem, D. E. *Nursing: Concepts of Practice.* New York: McGraw-Hill Book Co., 1971.

Peplau, H. E. *Interpersonal Relations in Nursing.* New York: G. P. Putnam's Sons, 1952.

Reynolds, P. D. *A Primer in Theory Construction.* Indianapolis: The Bobbs-Merrill Co., Inc., 1971.

Riehl, J. P., & Roy, C., Sr. *Conceptual Models for Nursing Practice.* New York: Appleton-Century-Croft, 1974.

Rogers, M. E. *An Introduction to the Theoretical Basis for Nursing Practice.* Philadelphia: F. A. Davis, 1970.

Roy, C., Sr. *Introduction to Nursing: An Adaptation Model.* Englewood Cliffs, New Jersey: Prentice-Hall, Inc., 1976.

Sellew, G., & Nuesse, G. J. *A History of Nursing,* 2nd Edition. St. Louis: C. V. Mosby Co., 1951.

Schlotfeldt, R. M. The significance of empirical research for nursing. *Nursing Research,* March/April, 1971, *20,* No. 2, pp. 140–142.

Shepherd, C. R. *Small Groups: Some Sociological Perspectives.* San Francisco, California: Chandler Publishing Co., 1964.

Susser, M. *Causal Thinking in the Health Sciences: Concepts and Strategies of Epidemiology.* New York: Oxford University Press, 1973.

Vaillot, M. C. Nursing Theory, levels of nursing, and curriculum development. *Nursing Forum,* 1970, *9,* No. 3, pp. 234–247.

Verhonick, P. J. *Nursing Research I* Boston: Little, Brown & Co., 1975.

Western Interstate Commission on Higher Education in Nursing, *Concept*

Formalization in Nursing Process & Product. Nursing Development Conference Group. Boston: Little, Brown & Company, Inc., 1973.

Woodruff, A. *Basic Concepts of Teaching.* San Francisco, California: Chandler Publishing Co., 1961.

Yura, H., & Walsh, M. B. *The Nursing Process,* 2nd Edition. New York: Appleton-Century-Crofts, 1973.

5
Literature Review

A review of relevant literature is important to research because the researcher needs to relate the proposed study to existing theory and to previous studies, and to develop sound hypotheses. This chapter explores the purposes of a literature review, methods of conducting one, and a way of presenting the results. All of these are illustrated with examples.

PURPOSES OF A LITERATURE REVIEW

When a student begins to consider a problem for possible investigation, the related literature should be reviewed. A literature review usually begins with a defined problem. As will be seen in Chapter 6, problem selection is most easily accomplished if the student considers the nature of the problem as defined in the literature. This chapter presents the literature review process for a defined problem. An example illustrating the literature review process for the topic of infantile autism is discussed. The problem was chosen as a result of a course on the special education of exceptional children. Material was presented in that course in such a manner that it became apparent that little was known about the disease. The student wished to learn about the educational outcomes for children with that condition. A literature review was undertaken to achieve that objective and to determine what answers had been discovered through research. Clearly, a defined problem that was identified in a classroom prompted this literature review. However, that is not always the case. Problems may be selected and defined as the result of a literature review alone.

Literature reviews conducted in search of topics assist students in clarifying ideas and in formulating specific problems that can be investigated by research methods. This process becomes understandable when one views the literature review, development of topics, and research as a " . . . slow and gradual process in which . . . one group of investigators builds on the works of others and, in turn, contributes their bit or bits, which may then serve as starting points for others" (Selltiz, Wrightsman, and Cook, 1976, p. 57). Thus, the student can understand the building blocks that provide the foundation for the construction of new theories. It is these blocks that form the basis for the development of a researchable topic.

To define a topic by first reviewing the literature, the student would initially identify a major subject of interest and then explore the blocks of the foundation supporting that subject. For example, if the area of pediatrics is selected, the student would next determine the specific aspects of pediatrics in which she or he is interested. To assist in that process, the student may ask: "Why do I care about pediatrics?" "Is it the setting (hospital, ambulatory clinic, community health clinic)?" "A particular disease (iron deficiency anemia, Hodgkin's disease)?" "A specific age group (infants, school age)?" Similar questions would be asked of any area of interest. Answers to such questions would define the topic by its relevant concepts and their attributes. These answers would be the building blocks of the topic. Once the area had been determined and the blocks identified, the student would review the literature related to that specific area. Further refinement of the topic occurs as the review progresses and more specific concepts are selected.

Refinement of the literature review can be explained using the following example: As a result of a community health nursing experience, the student developed an interest in pediatrics. The specific area was child abuse of first grade school-age children. The concept of abuse could uncover additional specific concepts such as mother-father-child relationships, financial status of the family, child performance in school, and attitudes and practices of the family toward child rearing. The student would review the sociological, psychological, financial, and educational literature. The sociological and psychological literature would reveal concepts related to family relationships and attitudes toward child rearing. The educational literature would be reviewed for the expected achievement levels of first-grade children. The economic literature could reveal the financial status of families with young children. It may be advisable to cross-reference the literature by comparing normal growth and development of children with the psychological literature for family attitudes toward young children. Another cross-reference that would be useful would be family attitudes (psychological) with financial status (economics). This may indicate to the student the existing relationships between poverty levels and their effects on family functioning in relation to children. This cross-referencing effort would unveil further concepts and would lead the student to a more complete review of the topic. Whether or not the topics proposed for review are important would depend primarily on the student's previous experience (was there evidence of child abuse in a family when the student gave care to the family during a home or clinic visit?) and on the student's common sense. If research studies are to be reviewed, the student also should evaluate the significance of the study findings to determine their relevance. Many related but extraneous concepts are likely to unfold.

Refinement of the child-abuse example is likely to include a large amount of apparently extraneous material. For instance, such information as the type of road surface (asphalt, dirt, cement, etc.) leading to the house of the family seems to be unimportant. However, if the road surface were a source of stress to the family, it could affect the family behavior toward the children. The student relies on past experience and common sense, attempting to gather as much pertinent information as possible in the topic refinement. This refinement process allows the investigator to change an undefined topic area (pediatrics) to a defined topic (child abuse). Obviously, this is accomplished through the publications of other researchers.

It should now be clear that the purpose of a literature review for any type of problem is to provide background knowledge about that problem and the development of a rationale for a proposed study. The student attempts to determine how the proposed study fits into the larger universe of related knowledge. Thus, it can be seen that previous studies will help to clarify the ideas and design of the student's proposed study (Cozby, 1977). The quantity of relevant literature available for review will depend on the popularity of the topic. A timely topic would include a greater number of publications than a relatively new topic with little popularity.

Time is required for the growth and development of new topics that are appropriate for research. Therefore, the first reason for conducting a literature review is to determine the extent to which the topic has been investigated. If it has been studied before, the findings may indicate areas in the proposed study that need to be redefined or rethought. Also, previous studies may assist the researcher in identifying areas for special attention in the proposed study, thereby preventing needless duplication (Lastrucci, 1967). A second reason for reviewing the literature is to permit the researcher to determine the extent to which the topic has been previously studied and what information has been found (Fox, 1976). Questions to consider are these: Are other studies consistent in their findings? Will expected findings from the proposed study enlarge or refute findings from other studies? Is the problem in the proposed study formulated differently than in previous studies? Do findings of previous studies justify the need for the proposed study (Batey, 1977)?

Finally, the literature should be reviewed so that the researcher can decide whether the proposed study would contribute to the relevant body of knowledge on the topic (Fox, 1976). Consideration should be given as to whether or not the proposed study is a part of a larger topic that has been studied or that is currently underway. If either of these conditions exist, the student would want to consider how the proposed study would relate to the larger topic. Is the proposed study only a replication of an earlier study; if so, what new knowledge would be gained and what advantage would be provided by the replication?

Based on the above considerations, the student will recognize that a literature review will provide some answers but also will raise questions. It assists in revealing the best avenues of approach for the proposed investigation (Lastrucci, 1967, p. 130). Further, it can provide an estimation of the success or the meaningful failure of the study (Fox, 1976, p. 285). Most important, a literature review will assist in developing the student's understanding of the topic. Based on these ideas and questions, the student then considers the methods that are used to conduct a literature review.

METHODS OF LITERATURE REVIEW

The Outline

A literature review should begin with the development of a clear outline of the subject to be studied. The outline is important to the student because it will encourage systematic, clear, and logical thought.

Figure 5-1 presents an outline that was developed for a research project. The project was to evaluate the weight loss of patients in a nurse-directed obesity clinic (Jones and Jenkins, 1973). This outline provided unity for the written literature review by allowing the researcher to identify gaps in coherence and by providing an overall emphasis for the study. The outline assisted in reinforcing the researcher's memory, and it provided continuity between inevitable interruptions. It can be seen that an outline plays a major role not only in organizing thinking but also in conducting the literature review related to the topic. A detailed process for developing an outline is to be found in Tichy (1966).

In planning the literature review, it is important to keep in mind the

I. Introduction
    A. Background
        1. Reports
            a. Nursing
            b. Medicine
            c. Clinic
    B. Purpose of study
II. The setting and the study plan
    A. Origin
        1. The problem
        2. Nursing intervention based on nursing diagnosis
    B. The actors
        1. Personnel involved
            a. Dietitian
            b. Psychologist
            c. Nurse
            d. Researcher
        2. The patients
    C. General considerations for planning
            a. Constraints
            b. Group approach
    D. Problems in working together
III. Final design of clinic study
    A. Number of patients
    B. Duration
    C. Roles of noninvolved staff
    D. Relationship to out-patient department
IV. Plan for assessment
    A. Objectives—major purpose
        1. Group
        2. Dietary
    B. Criteria for patient selection
    C. Constraints to patient selection
        1. Time
        2. Number of patients
        3. Drop-outs
    D. Criteria for success (outcome measures)
        1. Weight loss
        2. Knowledge
        3. Patient satisfaction
    E. Information gathering
        1. Baseline
        2. On-going
        3. Change indicators (posttest)
V. Summary
    Bibliography

Figure 5-1. Outline developed for an obesity clinic study.

time allocation proposed for conducting the study. The researcher would ask: "How much time should be allowed to review the literature?" The answer would depend on the complexity of the study. A complex study, for example, may be one that gathers data from international settings. A hypothetical example serves to illustrate this complexity. A study purpose is stated: "To determine the nursing needs of patients with the infectious disease tuberculosis (Tbc)." This condition is prevalent in five different countries. Care of patients with Tbc may be dependent on nurses with various educational preparations, countries with varied resources to meet the health needs of the patients and their families, and nurse investigators with different research aims. Conducting a literature review for such a project would involve the investigation of areas related to all of these considerations. This complex topic would require a detailed outline and literature review. Such a study would require many weeks, perhaps months, of work before its completion. However, the time allocation for the literature review of a student who is studying research in a classroom setting would be relatively short. The amount of time required for a literature review would also depend on the date set for study completion, the number of people involved in the data collection process, the time required for study review and for approval by faculty or agencies, and the need to obtain consent from proposed subjects. With a fully developed outline and a time table established, the student turns to the library for a search of the literature related to the topic.

The Library

A library search requires careful thought by the researcher about the topic under study. It must be remembered that the search should allow the student to place the problem in a larger universe. Two examples will clarify this process. Suppose a student wants to study the weight loss of 100 low-income obese patients who are cared for in the outpatient department of a hospital. Several specific diets designed to control weight gain would be used. The literature to be reviewed might include:

- Previous studies of obesity
- Economics of poverty
- Physiology of obesity
- Psychology of obesity
- Reducing diets
- Complications of weight loss

The second example is drawn from a literature review of infantile autism. Categories developed in that example related to the disease and included:

- Etiology
- Treatment
- Education
- Prognosis for recovery

After enumerating categories related to the problem, the student would then go to the library and begin the search for relevant references. If the student is using an unfamiliar library, the first person to consult would be the librarian. The librarian would describe the layout of the library so that the student would know where to locate the references. The librarian would answer questions related to the use of the library, such as what resources are available, where they are to be found and how they are used. Next, the student would become familiar with the library and its various procedures. There might be rules relating to a reserve book collection, interlibrary loans, special collections, copyright laws, and use of periodicals. Resources would include the card catalogue, photocopying services, and various computerized reference services.

Other Resources

There are many resources that are used for conducting a literature review. The major ones are the journals published by nursing organizations in which researchers report their investigations (Cozby, 1977). Some of these journals are related directly to nursing research, patient care, and to nursing administration. The student is directed to *Nursing Outlook,* May, 1978, pp. 325–329, for a list of the United States and Canadian indexes, dictionaries, abstracts, audiovisuals, directories, and bibliographies related to nursing. Other references related to specific health topics can be found with the help of the librarian or in the *Index Medicus.*

The *Index Medicus,* published monthly by the National Library of Medicine, is a guide to articles related to medical and health topics. It is indexed by both authors and subjects and contains references from more than 5,000 journals, approximately ten of which are nursing journals. Annual compilations of the monthly issues have been published since 1956. Whether a topic is familiar or unfamiliar to the student, this guide, which is clearly indexed and easy to use, is a good place to begin to identify relevant literature. The student should approach the *Index* with paper and pen in preparation for taking notes. Lined 3 × 5 file cards are useful for recording citations and notes. The notes should include not only the specific citations but also their titles.

Once a usable reference has been located, the student begins a critical review, taking notes while reading. For example, if the article was a research study, did the author present the study purpose, the material studied, the methods used, the data analysis, and the findings? How old is the study? Was anything missing? How relevant is the article to the problem? Was anything new found? Did it confirm previous studies? Chapter 15 will present more material on the process of critical reviewing in the form of critiquing articles. For the present purpose, the most important consideration for the student is the relevance of the article to the student's interest and the importance of its findings.

The student continues in this way to examine the individual articles identified by use of the *Index Medicus* or other references. The student would develop a relevant reference list based on the articles found in the *Index*. An example should clarify this process. Suppose the student is interested in reviewing the literature about the nursing care given to children who have been diagnosed as having infantile autism. The subject of "autism" would be sought in the *Index* to locate the material that has been published about that topic in various journals. The student would read those references, noting and reading any references listed at the end of each article that seemed relevant (Wandelt, 1970). This process would continue until the student had read or was familiar with most of the material on infantile autism.

Sometimes the specific word used by a student for labelling a problem is not found in the bibliographic reference. In that case, it is necessary to find a synonym or a broader word. For example, if "autism" were not found (which is unlikely), a student might look under "exceptional child" or "child, exceptional." It is also possible to explore additional bibliographic resources.

In recent years, computers have come into use to permit more extensive literature searches. One of these is known as Medlars, operated by the National Library of Medicine. This is a rapid computerized program for searching the literature related to a large number of health topics. Some large medical libraries have access to Medline, which produces a computer print-out list of citations on a specific topic. For this resource one usually must make an appointment through the librarian. The librarian will tell the student the amount of time needed to run the program, the methods used, the programming assistance needed, and the rapidity of retrieving the information. Results may be produced in the form of a print-out of citations. A fee for this service may be charged. Libraries in many universities have such a resource; however, the student is urged to begin a search with the *Index Medicus* or other printed bibliography, if for no other reason than to determine the best possible phrases for the intended request of the retrieval system.

Another source for the literature on a particular topic may be found in abstracts that are published by many professional fields. These are titles and very brief summaries of articles. Because there are so many of them, the student should consult a librarian about the appropriate abstract journal to use. Abstracts, although often too brief to be definitive, do help to identify articles that should be read in full. Abstracts should never be included as references in a literature review. Informative abstracts are found at the beginning of each article that is published in *Nursing Research* and in several other journals.

In conducting a literature review, the student should condense or abstract the relevant articles that were read. Then the student can read the material carefully, including the tables and footnotes, and take notes on important information for future use (Taylor, 1967).

The articles that are chosen for references should be grouped in accordance with the study outline into such categories as history, concept, methods, previous findings, and unanswered questions. When small file cards are used, it is easy to sort them into such categories. Some articles should be cross-referenced to two or more categories. In this way the literature review material is systematically organized for use in writing the research report. For a distinctive literature review, it is suggested that the student read all relevant literature, and read the original sources of any literature reviewed, not depending on their abstracts. In addition, he or she should take notes on the content of all the material reviewed (Beatty, 1973). Clearly, maintaining a record of all of that information requires organization of the materials.

Organization of Materials

In reviewing many pieces of literature, the student is wise to develop a system for organizing the information. This organization can begin with a review of the written notes based on the materials reviewed. This is easily accomplished using a matrix. A matrix is like a checkerboard in which several factors are interrelated in each article. In the infantile autism example, in which 60 studies were reviewed, the matrix had columns labeled Name of Investigator and Citation; Kind of Study, with two subcolumns (labeled Treatment and Observation); General Aims (Purpose); Number of Subjects (indicating age); Milieu, with two subcolumns labeled Day Care and Hospital; and the Results. The matrix was filled in as each article was read and notes taken so that the investigator could quickly summarize the relevant literature on infantile autism. An example of the format, using two of the 60 studies, is given in Table 5-1.

This type of format allows the student to summarize the 60 studies and coordinate the material. All of the treatment studies in hospitals can be clearly identified by focus of the study, number of subjects, general aims, and results. The treatment studies in day care centers can be identified similarly, as can descriptive studies in hospitals and descriptive studies in day care centers.

A matrix could be used for any type of study. With careful thought, the column headings could be changed to indicate, for example, the variables under study, the instruments used for data collection, or any other relevant aspects of the study. Such items would be entered under the Kind of Study heading. However, the student should develop a matrix that is specific for the study purpose and that meets the student's special needs. It can be said that any type of matrix is a useful tool for reviewing material from an organized format.

At the time that the notes are being organized, whether in a matrix format or not, the student should develop a reference list of the materials reviewed. References and the reader's notes can be recorded on index cards as illustrated below in Figure 5-2.

Figure 5-2 illustrates a method for documenting information on a file card. The student records the type, purposes, and general outcome of the study. Having such readily available summary information provides the student with the material necessary for a literature review.

Small study at the University of Cincinnati School of Nursing, where students evaluated their nursing instructors. Purpose of this pilot study was to:

1. Determine reactions of students and instructors to evaluation of instructors and of courses.
2. Determine when evaluation form should be used.
3. Collect information on variability and adequacy of the form used.
4. Determine the feasibility of using a specific evaluation procedure.

Response: Issue was controversial, but there was an apparent desire for students to participate in such evaluations in some way.

Figure 5-2. Notes of a literature review recorded on an index card. (From Mims, F., Students evaluate faculty, *Nursing Outlook,* July, 1970, *18* [7], pp. 53–55.)

Table 5-1. Sample Matrix Showing Two Research Studies

Name of Investigator and Citation	*Kind of Study*		General Aims	Number of Subjects	*Milieu*		Results
	Treatment	*Observation*			*Hospital*	*Day Care or Out-Patient*	
Cowan, P.A., et al, "Compliance & Resistance in the Conditioning of Autistic Children, An Exploratory Study." *Child Development* December, 1965, 36: 914-923.		Behavioral	To determine the amount of compliance and resistance in the conditioning of autistic children by asking them to choose red and square objects from a stimulus array	12 (ages 4–9 years)	X		Autistic children tend to be negativistic. They resisted the chores. Investigators felt that if compliance could be increased by training, paths would be opened for future psychometric testing and treatment
Coffey, H.S. & Wiener, L.L., *Group Treatment of Autistic Children*. Englewood Cliffs, N.J.: (Prentice-Hall, Inc.), 1967	Psycho-therapy		To determine the amount of improvement through the use of group treatment with autistic children	3–5 per group (5–12 years of age)		X	There was a trend toward improvement

The books by Treece and Treece (1977) and Turabian (1973) are useful guides for the preparation of a literature review.

PRESENTATION OF THE LITERATURE REVIEW

With a fully developed outline and the literature search completed, the student is ready to prepare the literature review in narrative form. The mode of presentation of the literature review is likely to vary depending upon its ultimate purpose. In any case, the purpose is to summarize what is already known about the topic or problem to be investigated.

The reasons for reviewing literature may be to satisfy requirements for education, publication, or funding. In educational settings, the reviews may be written as classroom assignments for research courses, master's theses, or doctoral dissertations. In such cases, the faculty members clearly outline the requirements. Some publications may not include a literature review section with their articles. In those instances, relevant material would be included as part of the article content. Study proposals submitted for funding tend to include literature reviews as a required part of the total packages. The format for any of these literature reviews is usually specified by each receiver; that is, faculty member, journal, or funding agency. For any of those purposes, the student should obtain information about the desired format and content before writing the literature review. It is suggested that the student initiate the literature review while the study protocol is being developed. In this way the major aspects of the literature would accrue and provide a good beginning for the final writing of the literature review. When the study protocol is completed, the student would begin writing the final literature review.

It is proper to begin any literature review with a statement of its objectives. For example, in a review for a study about physical and emotional needs of hospitalized patients, the beginning might be stated as follows: "All humans share a desire to have their needs met. Individuals vary, however, in their capacity to know their own needs and in the relative importance they give to different needs. Since the concept of need, factors affecting needs, and factors affecting perceptions of need are key elements in the study, the literature review discusses these points" (Williamson, 1976). The student would then follow this summary outline in the writing of the literature review.

After the statement of objectives, the student presents relevant material, using paraphrases as often as possible of any ideas discovered in the references. A large series of quotations is to be avoided, but an occasional quotation may be desirable. If the literature contains some ideas that are supportive of the thesis and others that do not support the thesis, those relevant ideas should be presented individually in sentence form. Citations can be presented at the end of a sentence. Using the patient-need example, a sentence might be written as "Relief from discomfort such as pain was discussed by Abdellah and Levine (1957), Newman (1966), and Rabkin (1973)." Or, a citation may become the subject of a sentence such as "Ingles (1960) stated that barriers to meeting patient needs were of a broad nature." The student would then describe briefly the factors that support the thesis and those that do not.

Care should be taken in choosing language for a literature review. Avoid the use of jargon! Lack of precision in the use of words may mislead the reader. The content and style of the literature review must receive attention for the consideration of readers, whether they are faculty, funding agencies, or students. Although there are no set rules regarding the time for the onset of a literature review, the review should show relationships to appropriate theories and to the development of hypotheses. It should demonstrate insightful thinking by the student. The literature review is a part of the foundation for the research study and should receive careful attention.

SUMMARY

This chapter has presented material related to the importance and processes of literature reviews for both defined and undefined problems. Areas stressed were the purposes of conducting a literature review and the methods for its development. Organization of materials was illustrated with the use of a matrix and file cards. Particular attention was given to the role of the library and its various resources. Last, a format for presenting the final review was discussed. It was shown that final reviews should reflect knowledge gained about the problem under study.

Students who have read and studied this chapter will know how to begin a literature review and what questions to ask for guidance in the use of resources. They will have attained an understanding of the purpose and role of a literature review in a research study. Further, these students will be able to identify the parts of a research problem that need a literature review. A review of the literature strengthens the development of the hypotheses to be tested in any proposed research study.

BIBLIOGRAPHY

Abdellah, F. G. and Levine, E. Polling patients and personnel, Part III. What personnel say about nursing care. *Hospitals,* December 1, 1957, *31,* No. 23, pp. 53–57.

Batey, M. Conceptualization: Knowledge and logic guiding empirical research. *Nursing Research,* September/October 1977, *26,* No. 5, pp. 324–329.

Beatty, W. K. Searching the literature comes before writing the literature. *Annals of Internal Medicine,* December 1973, *79,* No. 6, pp. 917–924.

Coffey, H. S., & Weiner, L. L. *Group Treatment of Autistic Children.* Englewood Cliffs, N.J.: Prentice-Hall, Inc., 1967.

Cowan, P. A., Hoddinoth, B. A., & Wright, B. A. Compliance & resistance in the conditioning of autistic children: An exploratory study. *Child Development,* December 1965, *36,* pp. 914–923.

Cozby, P. C. *Methods in Behavioral Research.* Palo Alto, California: Mayfield Publishing Co., 1977.

Fox, D. J. *Fundamentals of Research in Nursing,* 3rd Edition. New York: Appleton-Century-Crofts, 1976.

Ingles, T. Do patients feel lost in a general hospital? *American Journal of Nursing,* May 1960, *60,* No. 5, pp. 648–651.

Jones, Y. W., & Jenkins, L. A. A nurse-directed outpatient obesity clinic. *Hospitals,* November 16, 1973, *47,* No. 22, pp. 74–78.

Lastrucci, C. L. *The Scientific Approach.* Cambridge, Massachusetts: Schenkman Publishing Co., Inc., 1967.

Mims, F. Students evaluate faculty. *Nursing Outlook,* July, 1970, *18,* No. 7, pp. 53–55.

Newman, M. A. Identifying and meeting patients' needs in short-span nurse/patient relationships. *Nursing Forum,* 1966, *5,* No. 1, pp. 76–87.

Rabkin, M. T. The needs of patients. *New England Journal of Medicine,* May 10, 1973, *288,* No. 19, pp. 1019–1020.

Reference sources for nursing. *Nursing Outlook,* May, 1978, *26,* No. 5, pp. 325–329.

Selltiz, C., Wrightsman, L. S., & Cook, S. W. *Research Methods in Social Relations,* 3rd Edition. New York: Holt, Rinehart & Winston, 1976.

Taylor, S. D. How to prepare an abstract. *Nursing Outlook,* September 1967, *15,* No. 9, pp. 61–63.

Tichy, H. J. *Effective Writing,* New York: John Wiley & Sons, 1966.

Treece, E. W., & Treece, J. N. *Elements of Research in Nursing,* 2nd Edition. St. Louis: The C. V. Mosby Co., 1977.

Turabian, J. L. *A Manual for Writers,* 4th Edition. Chicago: The University of Chicago Press, 1973.

Wandelt, M. *A Guide for the Beginning Researcher.* New York: Appleton-Century-Crofts, 1970.

Williamson, Y. M. *Congruence between Nurses' and Patients' Perceptions of Patient Needs during Hospitalization.* The Johns Hopkins University, Doctoral Dissertation, 1976, p. 6.

6
Hypotheses Development

The goal of research is to test hypotheses; the outcome is to advance knowledge, test theories, or test models. Both the goal and outcome of research are dependent on the problem under investigation and the hypotheses to be tested. The purpose of this chapter is to present the process of hypotheses development. The chapter begins with the selection of the problem to study. The problem is the keystone for any hypotheses.

PROBLEM SELECTION

Hypotheses development begins with the problem or topic selected for investigation. A problem is something that seems wrong or raises questions. It can be described as the difference between the way things are and the way things should be. It is also a discrepancy or incongruence between two sets of facts (Diers, 1971). Selecting a problem for research purposes can be an eventful process for nurses in any health care setting.

The problems for study may stem from many interrelated sources. They may be found in the literature, various research reports, and a nurse's curiosity asking "I wonder why?" or "What would happen if?"

If the above suggestions are not fruitful, one can approach the problem selection with the use of an individual exercise. The following exercise has been used in a classroom setting: The students were asked to face the blackboard and think about what could be seen. They were then asked to consider the following questions: Is the blackboard attached and if so, how? What is its color and reflections of light? Does it have a chalk board? How much space does it occupy in terms of total wall space and total room space? What effects does room temperature have on it? What is its purpose? How often is it used, that is, what evidence is manifested of its use? What is its relationship to the rest of the building? Do different people see different things? The students were then asked to discuss their various answers to those questions. They quickly realized that more comprehensive observations evolved from the total group discussion than from their individual observations. Progressing through that exercise demonstrated to the students the need for a purpose ("Why are we doing this?"), and the importance of relationships (there would be no ceiling to the building if there were no walls or blackboard). The role of variables became clear when discussing room temperature, various effects of lighting, amounts of heat and amount of blackboard use. Progressing through that exercise demonstrated the need for a purpose, the importance of relationships, and the role of variables. Such an exercise conducted, whether by a group or on an individual basis, would help a person identify a problem to study and, at the same time, realize important aspects of research inquiry. However, no matter what type of source is used, that is, the literature, research reports, personal curiosity, or such a described exercise, the problem would arise from various personal considerations as well as certain social factors. The personal considerations may evolve from a person's value assignments and the availability of social support systems. These aspects should be recognized before the researcher makes a final selection of a problem.

Personal Considerations in Problem Selection

The selection of a problem for study may depend on the researcher's personal interest in or experience with a particular topic. This would be especially evident for a nurse caring for a group of patients with specific health problems, such as decubitus ulcers, obesity, or hypertension. For example, the idea for a research problem may originate with a hospital staff head nurse caring for patients with decubitus ulcers. The nurse realizes that many patients on the unit are experiencing a large number of skin problems. The nurse begins to question the effectiveness of the nursing care, the appropriateness of prescribed medications, and patients' abilities for self-care in turning without nursing assistance. The nurse would want to have answers to such questions as "How many patients equals a large number?" "What are the patients' rates of skin ulceration and healing?" and "What are her own skills as an attentive head nurse?" These questions could be answered through a scientific investigation. A researchable problem has been identified from the nurse's interest and personal experience.

Whether or not the nurse could conduct such a study may depend on certain social factors.

Social Factors in Problem Selection

Social factors or considerations may be an important aspect of the problem selection process. These factors may relate to the level of social prestige that a topic enjoys and thus the availability of support. Support may be in various forms, including agency agreement for the use of their setting, personal consent of individuals to participate as subjects, and financial aid for the conduct of the study.

One of the most important of these social considerations relates to financial support, without which the conduct of some research may not be possible. For example, topics that have been previously studied or are of a taboo nature may have little chance for funding outside the "home" agency. However, topics that are perceived (viewed) as innovative or needed by society would be more likely to receive financial support. Examples of these may be found in the social concerns with cancer prevention and introduction of health education into the baccalaureate nursing curriculum. Funding for investigation of these topics and many others comes from various sources, including the United States government, various foundations, and private individuals. Before seeking funds from any sources, the researcher must identify the problem to be investigated, its importance to the funder, and its relevance to society.

Problem Definition and Delineation

When a problem or topic has been selected to investigate, it must be defined and delineated. The definition is the foundation upon which the researcher builds the research project. Students may have learned that problem definition and problem delineation are used synonymously. However, professional investigators are likely to use the two terms to reflect different meanings. Problem definition involves defining the scope of the problem, whereas the aspects of the study are delineated. Based on the problem definition, items that dictate the extent and content of the investigation are then determined.

Some investigators view problem definition as the most difficult aspect of the research process. Clearly, it is central to the research endeavor and is composed of several factors that are delineated. First, the problem should be kept to a manageable size, that is, one that would comfortably fit into the time-frame established by the researcher.

Sample size, methods of data collection, and data analysis are some of the considerations.

Another factor to consider in the delineation of the problem is the relationship that the problem has with other concepts. It is important to consider the study's possible influence on existing concepts. For example, how does the patient's problem of fluid retention relate to the normal physiology of the body, patient stress due to difficulty in ambulating, or loss of appetite and its relationship to nutrition.

A third factor to consider in defining a problem addresses the notion of social utility. The researcher should be able to answer the *so what* question of the study. In other words, why conduct the study? What would the study accomplish for the agency, the subject, or a larger body of knowledge? There are several resources available to the research investigator in answering that question. Gaining that answer would depend on the researcher's knowledge about the problem, which could be obtained in many ways. In the decubitus ulcer example, the knowledge was gained through observations that resulted in wondering why. The head nurse observed the patients' conditions and wondered why these conditions existed. The researcher next would study the literature on the topic, disucss it with some experts, and then examine the relationships that became evident. The *so what* answer would begin to develop.

After a problem has been identified and defined, the researcher states the study purpose, which gives focus and direction to the study. The purpose determines the need for a solution to the research problem or to test a theory. The purpose should develop logically. Once the relationships are identified and a purpose has been stated, the researcher begins to define the concepts and develop hypotheses related to the problem.

Concepts: Operational Definitions

A major condition for constructing hypotheses concerns definitions of concepts used in the hypothesis. A concept is an abstraction. Definitions are labeling statements that indicate what each term means (Reynolds, 1971). To cite a hypothetical example, suppose a study purpose reads "To measure the length of time it takes for a patient to ambulate after suffering from a stroke leaving a left side paralysis." One hypothesis is stated: "The patient will feel more comfortable following ten minutes of ambulation." The *ten minute* aspect of the hypothesis is defined. It is measurable by the clock. However, the other words, *patient, more comfortable,* and *ambulation* must be operationally defined so that other investigators will have an understanding of their meanings. Each of those words would have a different meaning for each person asked. For example, Is the patient young, old, otherwise healthy? Who defines *comfortable* and by what criteria? Would the definition come from the patient, his nurse, a family member? What difference would that make? How much is more; that is, more than what? What is the denominator for analyzing the amount of more? This is, what are total possible amounts or the denominator of the measure? Similar questions would be raised over the word *ambulation*. Would ambulation require help; if so, how much and of what type? A cane, a walker, a person? Does ambulation mean first two steps, first walk across the room, how far? It quickly becomes evident that the hypothesis, as stated, is not clear or measurable. Operational definitions must be attached to the critical variables or factors so that they can be understood or so they can be rendered measurable.

Operational definitions indicate the procedures to be used in measurement. These definitions would be related to the study purpose. In the preceding example the patient may be defined as a 60-year old male experiencing his first hospitalization. State of comfortableness is defined as the patient and nurse report it; the patient and the nurse will report indicators of its existence, and it is measured by the patient's ability to sleep through the night without medication. Ambulation is operationally defined as "patient taking four steps without the aid of his nurse or a hand cane." These operational definitions would permit analysis of the hypothesis. Each concept has a built-in measurement tool in the form of indicators. The patient is measured by age, sex, and first hospitalization experience. Comfortableness is measured by the need for sleeping medication. If the amount of medication administered is an indication of the level of comfort, then the comfortableness is measured by inference. Ambulation is measured by the number of steps without the aid of a nurse, hand cane, or both.

DEVELOPMENT OF HYPOTHESES

When the researcher has selected a problem and identified and defined the concepts and study purpose, attention is turned to the development of hypotheses to test that purpose. In order to develop hypotheses, however, one must know what they are, where they come from, and how they are constructed. There are several ways to define a hypothesis. One definition is that a hypothesis is a statement that evolves from the problem and announces the relationship that the researcher expects to find between two or more items (variables). Another definition is that a hypothesis is a "proposition derived from a theory by deductive inference and which permits a test of empirical information" (Lastrucci, 1967). Either of these definitions can be used, but this text uses the first definition given. It is also important to note that different words may be used in the literature to mean hypotheses. These words may include "context," "law," "hunch" (Stephens, 1968). No matter which word is used, hypotheses function as guides to the type of data to be collected and to answers to the research questions. Hypotheses also determine the manner in which data can be most efficiently analyzed. To use hypotheses, however, it is necessary to understand their sources and methods for their construction.

Different types of research designs (see Chap. 7) have varying needs for hypotheses. However, in general, "factor- or situation-predicting" and "situation" or "factor-producing" investigations have hypotheses. A descriptive study (factor-isolating or factor-relating) of nominal data may not enjoy that status.

Sources for Hypotheses

Hypotheses may be generated from several sources. One of these sources is a hunch that comes from personal experience. This source would not necessarily provide assurance that the relationship of this study would be useful in other studies. However, it may be useful for inductive theory building or for contributing to a body of knowledge. Hypotheses may also arise from findings of other studies. These are not as limited as those arising from hunches, but they still may not be related to a larger body of knowledge or a theory. Finally, hypotheses may derive from an existing theory. To accomplish that derivation, one uses a process of deduction from theory and predicts that if certain conditions exist, certain results will follow. This helps to confirm a general theory and to strengthen the process of prediction. In developing hypotheses, the researcher should note the sources of the hypotheses and consider those sources in relation to the expected study outcomes. Does the researcher want to advance a new or existing theory, enrich a body of knowledge, or strengthen predictive ability about unknown or newly developed information? Once these questions are answered, the researcher constructs the hypotheses.

Construction of Hypotheses

Hypotheses must meet several conditions for their clear construction. First, each one should be expressed in a single sentence, using present-tense verbs. This prevents misunderstandings in their interpretations. Second, they should contain at least two variables that are under study. These variables are called the dependent and independent variables. The hypotheses may also reflect some uncontrolled variables. Clarifying the roles of the three kinds of variables in developing hypotheses is the second condition to meet for hypothesis construction. This permits understanding of the outcomes of hypothesis analysis.

As a third condition, the hypothesis must also serve as a guide for the kind of data to be collected. The ambulation example previously given makes this clear. However, some hypotheses may be constructed without apparent relationship to a study purpose. Suppose a purpose is stated as "To measure the number of times a patient in pain turns on his call light to request pain medications." An inappropriate hypothesis could say "Nurses spend most of their night shift time drinking coffee." Obviously, this is entirely unrelated to the study purpose. It is clear that hypotheses should be based on the definitions of the major concepts under study (e.g., pain, ambulation). Well constructed hypotheses contain proper syntax, appropriate variables, and clear definitions.

Variables in Hypotheses Construction

The variables are those items or factors that can and probably do vary in the systems of which they are units. There are three kinds of variables: dependent, independent, and uncontrolled variables.

The dependent variable is influenced or changed by the independent variable. An independent variable stands alone; it influences or changes the dependent variable. These two kinds of variables work together in a presumed cause-and-effect type of relationship or at least in some type of association (Cozby, 1977). Uncontrolled variables are those that the researcher cannot control. They are factors that exist but about which no data may be collected, or circumstances preclude manipulation. It is easy to understand that uncontrolled variables could have a great influence on study findings. An example will clarify the relationship among the three kinds of variables.

A researcher conducts a study to investigate the relationship between nurses' grade point averages (GPAs) and their admission to graduate schools. The GPA scores are the independent variables for any given person at a point in time (they do not change) and the admissions are the dependent variables (they do change). Admissions would depend on the GPA scores. The uncontrolled variables would include factors such as the events that might have influenced a low GPA score, sudden changes in school admission policies, or the health status of the person during her or his previous educational experience. Unless these variables were included as part of the hypothesis, they should be viewed as uncontrolled or confounding, and they would influence the research findings.

Another example of variables can be shown in the relationship between drug abuse and crime rates. Crime rates may be associated with the type and amount of drug used by the study subject. The uncontrolled variables could include any event(s) affecting either the intake of drugs or an unknown reason for commiting a crime. These factors should be considered in relation to the specific study purpose and hypotheses. In this way findings could be clearly interpreted. With variables identified, the researcher considers the types of hypotheses.

Research and Null Hypotheses

Two types of hypotheses are used in research studies. They are the research hypothesis (signified as H_R) and the null hypothesis (signified as H_0). Nurse researchers tend to rely more on the H_R in conducting their studies. However, the hypotheses are interrelated. This section presents both types, showing their relationship. They are illustrated with simple hypothetical examples.

Research Hypotheses

Research hypotheses (H_R) are used in the applied sciences as program evaluations, data collection, tool development, and so on. This type of hypothesis is one that predicts a positive or negative relationship among the variables under study (Blalock, 1972). It states that there is a difference among variables, conditions, or events, and in what manner they differ. The following hypothetical example is used to illustrate the research hypothesis.

A nurse investigator wonders about the distribution of pediatric nurse practitioners (PNPs) in the southern states of Florida, Georgia, South Carolina, North Carolina, Virginia, and Maryland. This wondering is developed into a study rationale and purpose. The nurse plans a random selection of PNPs from the six states. The rationale and study purpose would support the following research hypothesis: "There are 35% more pediatric nurse practitioners employed in hospital settings than in public health settings in the southern states." The two variables are the PNPs (dependent) and employment settings (independent). Uncontrolled variables might include such factors as reason for job selection. The difference (more) and its magnitude (35%) are defined and measurable. A discussion of the findings would be meaningful to most interested investigators. If appropriate, the researcher may wish to develop subhypotheses for the overall study hypotheses. Such action would result in one hypothesis for each of the six southern states. It might be stated as "In Florida there are more PNPs employed in hospital settings than in public health settings." Testing the six alternative hypotheses would provide answers to the research question for each state as well as a more accurate account of the distribution of PNPs by work settings. Also, it could provide information about the ratio of PNPs to nurse practitioners (all types) by setting. This may vary by state. The researcher would be able to identify those states with high percentages of PNPs working in hospitals or where PNPs are overrepresented. Perhaps, if appropriate, the researcher would present recommendations, such as for administrative and educational changes, in an attempt to alleviate problems in areas underserved by pediatric nurse practitioners. Careful attention would be given to any uncontrolled variables. Obviously, recommendations would depend on the study purpose and would be based on all of the variables being studied.

Null Hypothesis

A null hypothesis is discussed using the PNP distribution problem. This type of hypothesis is used for testing, stating that there is no difference between the mean of the variables under study and the mean of the population from which they were drawn. The underlying assumptions for its use are as follows: 1) populations sampled are the same; in this example all of the PNPs are the same; and 2) sampling was random (Blalock, 1972). Chapter 8 discusses assumptions and their importance for the null hypothesis as well as for sampling.

Based on the PNP problem, the researcher can develop a null hypothesis that is stated as "There is no difference in the number of PNPs employed in hospitals versus public health settings in the southern states." It is hypothesized that the population of nurses in the two employment settings is the same. Whether the null hypothesis is accepted or rejected, the researcher cannot present a general discussion regarding underlying reasons. The investigator has only the evidence of the statistical analysis upon which to base that decision.

In statistically analyzing the null hypothesis, the investigator should note whether differences are real, or the product of imprecise data collection instruments or improper analysis. Inferential statistics used in their analysis (see Chap. 13) indicate how much of the difference is due to chance and provide evidence for acceptance or rejection; in other words, whether or not the hypotheses are probably true statements.

There is no established number of hypotheses that must be used in a study (Fox, 1976). The amount would depend on the complexity of the problem under study. A complex study is likely to have several hypotheses, with many subhypotheses relating to each one of them. It is important to realize that every hypothesis must be tested and finally reported. Once data are collected using either the research or the null hypotheses, they are statistically analyzed. The statistical analyses provide evidence for the acceptance or rejection of the hypotheses.

Testing Hypotheses

With hypotheses developed and data collected, the researcher is ready to consider which statistical tests are appropriate. In order to test hypotheses, the researcher must answer certain questions about the hypotheses.

The first question to answer is "What are the reasons for analyzing the data?" In other words, what does the researcher plan to learn? What is the type of relationship that has been established through the hypothesis?

A second question to answer is "What are the variables under study?" Independent, dependent, and uncontrolled variables have been presented. These variables should receive statistical attention.

Third, the researcher may wish to determine the scale of measurement that the data assume, "Is it nominal, ordinal, interval, or ratio?" (See Chap. 10 for a full discussion of these scales.) Once those questions have been answered, the researcher plans the type of statistic to use.

The central limit theorem is a good place to begin determining the type of statistic to use. Based on that theorem, the critical regions for the amount and direction of hypothesis acceptance are determined.

Critical Regions in Testing Hypotheses

In testing hypotheses, it is important to give the statistical evidence of their acceptance or rejection. Before data analysis, the researcher sets the level at which the hypothesis will be accepted with the minimal error. This level is expressed as a P value or alpha or the percent chance of being incorrect. In nursing research, a P value is often set at 5%, meaning that 5% of the time or less the findings may be due to chance. In other words, the probability that these findings are due to chance is less than 5%. This is written as $P < .05$, and it is stated as 95% of the time these findings are considered to be true. The researcher accepts the hypotheses. The statistical value may appear on the negative side of the normal curve. This would be true if the hypothesis were stated indicating a negative effect or outcome. In that case, the P value would be P = < − .05 and, as before, it is said that 95% of the time the findings would be true. Clearly, that would apply for the negative side of the normal distribution. See Chapter 12 for a presentation of the normal distribution.

Errors in Testing Hypotheses

In setting a critical region for acceptance of a hypothesis, there is a chance of making errors. These are known as alpha (P) and beta errors. An alpha error is also called a type I error. It is one that calls something false when it is true.

Type I errors are based on statistical information, as was just described. This type of error is made when a statistical difference is labeled real (significant) when it is due to chance. A true hypothesis could be rejcted. For example, if it is statistically stated that a variable called A is true, then the variable called B will probably be true, too. However, it must be admitted that variable B may be false when A is true. If A is rejected whenever B is false, we run the risk of rejecting a true hypothesis. Something is called false when it is real. In other words, a difference is labeled as significant (real) when it is due to chance. It can be said that the smaller the risk of the alpha error, the greater the probability of the beta error.

A beta, or type II, error is based on logical reasoning. This can be compared to the statistical reasoning underlying the type I error. A type II error is logically stating that something is real when it, in fact, is false. For instance, if it is stated that theory A leads to consequences B, it could not be said that A *must* be true. B may be true for other reasons. For example, suppose a hypothesis is stated that "nursing students with A averages in the medical clinical area would pour more precise dosages of medication for their patients than do students with D averages." Although that seems logically correct, it may not be true for many reasons unrelated to the students' educational achievements. Perhaps their level of precision is related to the expertise of the faculty responsible for their learning experience or their need to leave the clinical area for a meeting. Although the statement seems logically sound, accepting it as a hypothesis could result in the commission of a beta error. The precision related to the pouring of medication may not be related at all to students' educational achievement. Such a statement could result in the error of failing to reject a hypothesis or statement when it actually is false.

The relationship of type I and type II errors to decisions to accept or reject hypotheses is illustrated in Figure 6-1. The rows represent the decisions made on the basis of particular observations in the sample.

		HYPOTHESIS	
		Actually True	*Actually False*
DECISION	To accept	(1) Correct	(2) β error or type II error
	To reject	(3) α error or type I error	(4) Correct

Figure 6-1. Relationship of types of errors and outcome of hypotheses. (Dixon, W.J., and Massey, F.J. *Introduction & Statistical Analysis,* 3rd. Edition. New York: McGraw-Hill Book Company, 1969. Reprinted with permission.)

The columns represent the truth or falsity of hypothesis. Correct decisions are in cells 1 and 4. In cell 1, a true hypothesis is accepted; in cell 4, a false hypothesis is rejected. Cell 2 is an incorrect decision because the true hypothesis was rejected. Cell 3 is an incorrect decision because the false hypothesis was accepted. Decisions whether or not to accept a hypothesis are statistically based. The reader is urged to refer to Dixon and Massey (1969) and Chapter 13 of this book for further discussion of errors.

Testing hypotheses is the foundation for scholarly reporting of research findings. Researchers must be aware of the various factors involved in the testing procedures so that the findings will have meaning to other investigators.

SUMMARY

This chapter has presented an overview of problem selections with emphasis on personal and social considerations as well as the definition and delineation of problems. Particular emphasis has been on the operational definitions of concepts. The properties, formulation, and functions of hypotheses were presented. Sources, types, and testing of hypotheses were discussed, indicating the process and importance of each topic. Relevant examples for each of these topics were given. The chapter should be viewed as an initial course of action to take in the process of hypotheses development.

BIBLIOGRAPHY

Blalock, H. M. *Social Statistics.* New York: McGraw-Hill Book Company, 1972.

Cozby, P. C. *Methods in Behavioral Research.* California State University, Fullerton: Mayfield Publishing Co., 1977.

Diers, D. Finding clinical problems for study. *Journal of Nursing Administration,* November/December 1971, *1,* No. 6, pp. 15–18.

Dixon, W. J., & Massey, F. J. *Introduction & Statistical Analysis,* 3rd Edition. New York: McGraw-Hill Book Company, 1969.

Fox, D. J. *Fundamentals of Research in Nursing,* 3rd Edition. New York: Appleton-Century-Crofts, 1976.

Lastrucci, C. L. *The Scientific Approach: Basic Principles of the Scientific Method.* Cambridge, Massachusetts: Schenkman Pub. Co., Inc. 1967.

Reynolds, P. D. *A Primer in Theory Construction.* New York: The Bobbs-Merrill Co., Inc., 1971.

Stephens, W. N. *Hypotheses & Evidence.* New York: Thomas Y. Crowell Co., 1968.

Part 3

THE RESEARCH DESIGN

Part 3 contains four chapters that provide the basic information needed to conduct research. Chapter 7 describes three types of research designs: descriptive, experimental, and quasi-experimental. Measurement scales, measurement errors, reliability, and validity are presented in Chapter 8. With that background, the reader is prepared for a variety of sampling techniques, explained in Chapter 9. This chapter includes definitions, concepts, and various sampling procedures. Probability, nonprobability, and sample size are stressed, and attention is given to nonsampling errors. Chapter 10 discusses the various instruments used to collect data. The chapter begins with an overview of methods of data production, including questionnaires and interviews. Special attention is paid to rating and scaling procedures. The reader is instructed in the selection of data collection tools. Chapter 11 introduces the topic of questionnaires. The emphasis in this chapter is on types of questionnaires, methods of administering questionnaires, problems related to informed consent, and response rates. How to construct a structured questionnaire is explained by an example. Upon completion of Part 3, the student should be prepared for the discussion of the analysis and reporting of collected research data presented in Part 4.

7
Types of Research Design

Cheryl S. Alexander

One of the most critical decisions a researcher must make is the selection of an appropriate design for a study. This choice is important because research designs serve as overall plans for making observations and collecting, organizing, and analyzing information. Basically, designs are blueprints for conducting research. Each design includes a set of rules or requirements that assist the researcher in making decisions about what kinds of phenomena should be observed, how best to make the observations, and what analysis strategies are most appropriate for testing relationships among phenomena.

This chapter describes and explains various types of research designs and their uses. Specific designs frequently used by nurse researchers are presented and discussed.

PURPOSES OF RESEARCH DESIGNS

The overall objective of any research design is to give the researcher maximum control over the study environment and over factors or variables. Research designs suggest ways in which the research can make the conditions under which information is collected approximately the same for every participant in the study. Well-conceived research designs increase the researcher's confidence that the findings are a valid representation of what occurs in the world.

For example, the student is asked by the Director of Nursing Services to evaluate the impact of primary nursing on patients' perceptions of nursing care. First, the student would identify several methods of nursing care organization. It is known that patients' satisfaction with nursing care can be affected by a variety of factors (e.g., type of patients on the unit or work load of the nursing staff) other than the method of nursing care organization. Furthermore, since the aim is to evaluate the impact of primary nursing on patient satisfaction, a second step would be to measure satisfaction on several units that have similar types of patients and nursing staff but that use a method of nursing care other than primary nursing.

In this example, the *purpose of the study* is to evaluate the impact of primary nursing on patients' perceptions of nursing care, and the *nature of the problem* is a comparison of primary nursing with some other form of nursing care organization. Both the purpose of the study and the nature of the problem suggest a design that uses two comparable groups and measures patient satisfaction with specific aspects of nursing care for each group over a predetermined time period. Note that the selection of a study design will not indicate which phenomenon should be investigated (method of nursing care organization) nor how the study groups should be selected (specific criteria for making the two groups comparable). It also does not specify what statistical techniques should be used for analyzing the data. However, the design does suggest a framework in which to make these decisions. Since design decisions stem directly from the purpose of the study and the nature of the research problem under investigation, it is important that a researcher have a well-defined purpose and a clearly formulated study question before selecting any research design. Therefore, good research is based on a well-conceived and carefully implemented research design. A research design provides a framework for selecting variables, study populations, and analysis strategies. The decision to choose one research design rather than another is directly related to 1) the purpose of the study and 2) the nature of the research problem.

LEVELS OF RESEARCH

Research studies may assume several different forms depending on the purpose of the study. Selltiz, Wrightsman, and Cook (1976) describe three broad types of research studies that can be viewed as representing "pure" forms of research resting on a continuum from problem formulation to hypotheses testing. These forms are formulative or exploratory, descriptive, and experimental. Seldom do research studies in the real world cluster neatly in one of these well-defined levels. Additionally, studies may have a descriptive phase and then move to a hypotheses testing phase as theoretical and methodological knowledge advance.

Although clear-cut distinctions cannot be made between various types of research studies, it is useful to examine briefly each level of research.

Formulation or Exploratory Studies

Formulation or exploratory studies represent a preliminary level of research. As suggested by their titles, these studies explore areas of inquiry that lack theoretical development. These studies identify research questions, clarify concepts, and construct hypotheses for testing at a later stage. Exploratory studies are useful when a researcher has identified an area of interest but finds that little is known about it. In this situation, an exploratory study can aid in concept formation and theory development. Selltiz, et al. (1976) suggest several other functions of exploratory research: the establishment of priorities for future research, collection of information about the practical possibilities of carrying out a research study in a real life setting, and establishing the need for research in a particular area by tapping the opinions of experts in the field.

An example of exploratory research is the following. Nurses working in a prenatal clinic are interested in knowing why some pregnant women register early in their pregnancy (first trimester) while others register late (third trimester). An initial step in this investigation would be to survey existing literature regarding the characteristics of women who choose prenatal care. It is fair to assume, at least initially, that the timing of prenatal registration has been previously examined. A thorough literature review will save time and energy in the long run because it is easier to build upon the work of others in formulating a research question than to "re-invent the wheel."

Based on the literature review, the nurses may want to describe systematically their two groups of clinic registrants. A chart review will help characterize certain sociodemographic and background features of these women, for example, age, parity, and marital status, but may do little to identify reasons for seeking or not seeking early prenatal care. For this kind of data, an interview or questionnaire might be useful. The interview or questionnaire would include both structured questions asking for specific information and open-ended questions designed to allow the patient to make whatever comments she feels are relevant. By categorizing responses to the questionnaire or interview and combining this information with the descriptions obtained from the chart review, it is likely that the nurses can formulate several research questions worthy of subsequent study.

Sometimes the objective of an exploratory study is to determine research priorities. Here, an *experience survey* may be helpful. The purpose of an experience survey is to gain insights into what should be the most important research questions addressed in a particular area. Respondents for such a survey are selected based on their competence and their work experience in the area of interest. Assume that the interest is in examining the adoption of nursing innovations (e.g., use of nurse-midwives in hospital settings). From a review of the literature, the researcher has compiled a list of nursing innovations that he or she thinks would be important to assess, but some external validation is needed. By surveying people with experience in hospital nursing administration, education, and clinical practice, the completeness of the list can be evaluated as well as the relative importance of each nursing innovation in the real world. This information is exceedingly helpful in deciding which nursing innovations should be given research priority and how they should be defined and measured. Also, a panel of experts can provide information about the practical aspects of conducting such a study. They can answer such questions as: What clinical facilities should be used? Which ones are likely to cooperate? Who should be approached to gain access to a site? What obstacles are anticipated in carrying out the study, and how might these be best surmounted? The answers to these kinds of questions can make a real difference as to whether a study operates smoothly or runs into road blocks.

It is important to remember that exploratory studies represent preliminary research efforts. They are designed to raise questions, not to provide empirical answers. They cannot assess cause-effect relationships, but they can formulate hypotheses about such relationships suitable for testing in more carefully controlled studies.

Descriptive Studies

Investigators are not in total agreement as to what constitutes descriptive research. Distinctions between exploratory and descriptive studies are frequently unclear, particularly when comparisons are made between elaborate exploratory studies and simple descriptive designs. Some of the confusion can be eliminated by remembering that the major way to differentiate among research studies is to examine the *aim* or purpose of the study.

Descriptive studies represent detailed accounting, either qualitative or quantitative, of a population, situation, or event. In their pure form, descriptive studies differ from exploratory studies in several ways. They require a well-formulated research question, a defined study population, and some clearly delineated measurement of the phenomenon of interest. Using the previous prenatal care example, a researcher might ask if women with complicated labor and delivery experiences in their previous pregnancies are *more* or *less* likely to seek early prenatal care. In this example, there is a research question, yet no presumption is made as to the direction of the relationship between past labor and delivery experiences and prenatal care registration. The question does not say that past pregnancy complications *lead to* early prenatal registration. Because they lack appropriate controls, descriptive studies cannot test hypotheses nor explain or predict relationships. However, these studies can make assessments of relationships between phenomena based on accumulated information. In this way, descriptive research is useful for planning and program evaluation.

Descriptive studies are relatively simple to conduct. The first step in the above example is to define the purpose of the study and to formulate a study question, which could be stated as follows: Is there an association between the timing of prenatal care registration and previous labor and delivery complications? Second, terms used in the study must be operationally defined. These would include pregnancy complications and prenatal care registration.

Operational definitions assist the researcher in establishing criteria for selecting a study population and for collecting data. In this proposed study, two samples of women in the prenatal clinic would be chosen: a group of early registrants (< 24 weeks) and a group of late registrants (> 36 weeks). Data would be collected from clinic records on the background characteristics of each group of women. This assumes that information about past labor and delivery experiences is available and is accurately recorded in the medical records.

After the data are collected, tabulations are made of the number of women with labor complications for early and late registrant groups. The researcher might want to cross tabulate labor complications with other variables such as parity, which might explain an observed difference between early and late registrants. Cross tabulation is a useful analysis strategy in assessing whether any difference between two study groups can be attributed to the effects of variables other than the ones of primary interest to the study. In this example, differences in labor and delivery complications may be attributed to differences in parity rather than differences in registration. Women at greater parity levels are more likely to have had labor and delivery complications because they have had more pregnancies. By comparing the proportions of women with labor and delivery complications in the early and late groups by their parity level, the researcher treats parity as if it were a constant. The proportion of women with labor complications at parity two who are in the early registrant group are compared with the proportion of women with complications at the same parity level who registered late in their current pregnancy. Parity no longer varies for the two groups of registrants, thus its influence on labor and delivery complications is eliminated. Other variables thought to influence labor and delivery complications can be examined in the same systematic way.

The use of operational definitions, criteria for selecting a study population, and analysis strategies gives descriptive research greater precision and accuracy in assessing relationships between phenomena than is possible to obtain in exploratory studies. When the purpose of the study is to advance knowledge or to test causal hypotheses, an experimental research design is required.

Experimental Research

An experiment is a scientific investigation, the major purpose of which is to explain relationships among phenomena. Experimental research represents the ideals of scientific inquiry, that is, prediction and explanation. A better understanding of the world can be accomplished by predicting the occurrence of phenomena and knowing why they occur. Descriptive and exploratory studies give us the ability to describe and examine relationships among phenomena, but only experimental studies are powerful enough to permit us to draw causal inferences about these relationships. The concept of causality implies both prediction and explanation.

Selltiz, et al. (1976) state that often a causal relationship is thought to be a single event leading to a single outcome. In reality, causal relationships are far more complex, frequently involving several events contributing to the occurrence of an outcome. The concept of causality is controversial. Some researchers take the position that, since a causal relationship can only be inferred and never be demonstrated conclusively, the concept has little practical value and should be abandoned. Other researchers believe that without the notion of causality, scientific knowledge cannot be advanced, since, in part, knowledge is achieved through the systematic testing of hypotheses. Thus, it can be said that the concept of causality serves as the primary basis for experimental research. Characteristics of experimental research, such as randomization, experimental manipulation, and the use of control groups, reflect ways of gathering evidence to make causal inferences about observed relationships.

CRITERIA FOR CAUSAL RELATIONSHIPS

Selltiz, et al. (1976) have identified three criteria for inferring a causal relationship: concomitant variation, temporal ordering of variables, and evidence that rules out other possible causal factors. These criteria are best met by experimental designs.

Concomitant Variation

Concomitant variation is the extent to which the independent and dependent variables occur together in the hypothesized direction. Let us assume that it is hypothesized that group therapy (independent variable) reduces the length of hospitalization (dependent variable) for alcoholic patients. As an initial step, a researcher would examine the hospital records of alcoholic patients who had group therapy and those who did not. If in the group of patients who experience short hospitalizations, it is found that a greater proportion of patients had group therapy (80%) than had some other form of therapy (20%), some evidence for concomitant variation would be provided. This one observation is not sufficient to *prove* that group therapy causes shorter hospitalization, because factors other than the type of treatment (e.g., age, sex of patient) could have produced similar findings. It does, however, suggest that the hypothesis is worthy of further investigation.

Time Order

By definition, a phenomenon can only be considered causal if it *precedes* the observed outcome. This temporal ordering of phenomena constitutes the second criterion for inferring a causal relationship. Returning to the previous example, the patients' participation in group therapy must have preceded their discharge from the hospital in order for group therapy to be considered as a causal factor. In this example, it is easy to determine which event came first. However, frequently the ordering of events is not as clearly distinguishable. For instance, if a large number of people who attended a luncheon appeared in the emergency room with nausea and vomiting, it would be important to determine which people suffered the digestive distress *before* and which people became ill *after* the luncheon. If the digestive symptoms appeared after eating, then an investigator would want to assess what foods or beverages were consumed at the luncheon. If the distress occurred before the luncheon, the luncheon could not be considered as the source of the vomiting and nausea. Temporal ordering provides additional supporting evidence for the existence of a causal relationship; but, like concomitant variation, it cannot prove causality. Again, other factors must be considered. These might include previous exposure to Asian flu, which might account for the digestive distress.

Elimination of Competing Explanations

In order to infer causality, an investigator must systematically rule out other possible causes of the observation. These other factors are often called competing explanations. They represent alternative ways of explaining why a phenomenon occurs.

To return to the alcohol unit example, it was observed that a greater proportion of patients who had experienced group therapy had shorter hospital stays on the alocholic unit than patients treated by some other means. Furthermore, group therapy treatment preceded the patients' discharge from the hospital. These two observations suggested that group therapy may result in shorter hospitalization for patients on this particular alcoholic unit. But other factors might explain shorter hospitalization. Suppose it was found that among those patients with shorter hospitalization, a greater proportion were under 25 years of age. Perhaps it is the patients' youth rather than the type of treatment received that contributed to the length of their hospitalization. Or suppose it was found that more men than women were represented in the shorter hospitalization group. Again, the sex of the patient could be considered a competing explanation for the shorter hospital stay.

These competing explanations must be eliminated if one is reasonably to infer that group therapy produces or causes shorter hospitalization. Competing explanations can be eliminated by design or by statistical controls. Throughout this discussion the term *infer* has been used when discussing causality. One can only infer causal relationships, since it is impossible to know all the factors that contribute to the occurrence of an outcome. Investigators might neglect to consider some factor associated with the independent variable (group therapy) that influences the outcome (length of hospitalization). Thus, although concomitant variation, temporal ordering, and elimination of competing explanations provide a basis for inferring causality, they are not grounds for *proof*.

EXPERIMENTAL DESIGNS

Designs for true experiments are far more rigorous than those designs used in exploratory or descriptive research. Since the purpose of experimental research is to *test* hypotheses, experimental designs are blueprints for collecting evidence for inferring causal relationships. The important characteristic of experimental research is *control.* The researcher seeks to maximize the effects of the independent or causal factor on some specific outcome while minimizing the effects of other extraneous or unwanted factors. The notion of control is introduced into the study design largely through the use of manipulation, randomization, and comparison groups.

Experimental Manipulation

In an experimental study, the researcher provides evidence for concomitant variation by manipulating the independent variable and then observing the effect of this manipulation on an outcome. Simply put, the researcher compares both groups on some measured outcome to see if the treatment or intervention had an effect. For example, in testing a hypothesis that group therapy reduces hospital stay, the researcher creates two groups of patients who share many of the same characteristics (e.g., age, sex, past history of alcohol problems). One group receives group therapy while the other group receives whatever treatment is currently in use on the unit. After a predetermined time period, the discharge records of both groups of patients are compared. If the researcher finds that a greater proportion of patients who had group therapy had shorter hospital stays, evidence that group therapy and reduced hospitalization are related has been provided. In this example, the researcher controls the causal factor by deliberately varying subjects, exposure to it. The ability to vary exposure is a principle characteristic of a true experiment.

In basic research, it is possible to manipulate the independent variable with relative ease; however, in applied research areas, such as nursing, ethical protection of human subjects often precludes variable manipulation. For example, a nurse who wants to evaluate the effectiveness of dietary teaching on diabetic patients' ability to plan meals that meet their insulin requirements would not be able purposely to provide dietary instructions for one group of patients while deliberately withholding information from another group. The nurse researcher might choose to compare effectiveness of a teaching method by comparing it with an existing method.

Alternatively, the nurse could search for a group of patients who for one reason or another did not receive any dietary information and compare their meal planning with a comparable group of diabetics who received diet teaching. This latter case constitutes a *natural experiment,* one in which exposure to the independent or treatment variable differs but is not under the control of the researcher.

Randomization

As a way of making the patient groups comparable, randomization, or random assignment, is used. Random assignment means that each patient on the alcohol unit at the time of the study had an equal chance of being assigned to either the experimental or therapy group or to the control or regular treatment group. This procedure helps reduce the possiblity that factors other than the treatment method would affect hospitalization. In other words, randomization helps to eliminate competing explanations for the hypothesized causal relationship by creating equivalent groups.

If age were related to length of hospitalization and all patients under 25 years of age were included in the experimental group, it would be difficult to determine if changes in hospital stay were due to the treatment intervention or because young patients tend to stay in the hospital for shorter periods of time. If, however, all the young patients appeared in the control group, a finding of no difference in length of hospitalization between experimental and control groups would be misleading. Perhaps the youth of the patients in the control group is reducing their length of hospitalization, thus balancing out the effects of group therapy in the experimental group. A real difference would be observed if each group had a similar age distribution.

The key factor here is the relationship of age to hospital stay. In this study, age is a known extraneous variable; that is, it is known that age influences length of hospitalization. Since the researcher is not interested in studying age, its effect on hospitalization must be controlled. There may be other patient characteristics, like age, that will influence length of hospital stay. These factors may be unknown. Nevertheless, their impact must be taken into account in order to have confidence in the genuineness of the findings. Randomization helps eliminate competing explanations for observed relationships between independent and dependent variables by equalizing the effects of other known and unknown factors.

Since randomization operates on the principles of chance, it does not always succeed in producing equal groups. This is particularly true if the number of subjects in the study is small. If there were ten alcoholic patients on the unit, five under the age of 25 and five who were over 25 years of age, by chance alone the five younger patients might be assigned to the group therapy treatment. Given this situation, it would be impossible to separate the treatment effects from age effects on length of hospitalization. The effectiveness of randomization as a means of control increases as the number of study subjects increases.

The process of randomization is a simple procedure. In the above example, the researcher could record the names of the ten patients on slips of paper, put the slips into a hat, fishbowl, or some other container, and then draw names. The first five names drawn would be assigned to the experimental or group therapy group and the second five to the control or standard treatment group. Flipping a coin to determine group membership is another simple way of randomizing subjects. It is predetermined that if the coin comes up heads, the subject is assigned to the experimental group; if tails, the subject goes to the control group. Obviously, these groups could be reversed.

Clearly, these strategies are impractical for large numbers of subjects. Researchers frequently use a table of random numbers to assist them in making group assignments. Random number tables often appear in the appendices of statistics textbooks. Using digits 0 to 9, these tables are constructed so that each number has an equal chance of following any other number. This construction allows the researcher to select numbers in any direction without fear of bias.

In the alcohol therapy example, the randomization process using a random number table is as follows. First, all of the patients on the alcohol unit would receive a number between one and ten. Next, a procedure would be determined for drawing random numbers from the table. For instance, it might be decided that after a random start, the first five numbers would be selected by moving to the right across the row. It is important that procedural decisions be made prior to drawing numbers, particularly in a large study where several individuals are involved in selecting study participants. Since a random number sequence can be generated by moving in any direction in the table, it is not the direction itself that is important but that everyone involved in drawing numbers follow the same procedure.

To demonstrate how random numbers are drawn, consider Table 7-1. The circled number represents our starting point and the arrows indicate the direction we will move to select numbers. A starting point is chosen by having someone close his or her eyes and point to part of the table, or by using a computer to generate the starting number. Next, we move along the row to the right looking for the first two-digit number that falls between 01 and 10. The first number we come to that meets the criterion is 0215. Looking at the list of patients, it is found that John D. has been assigned 02. He becomes the first member of the experimental group one. Moving along the row, the next number is

Table 7-1. Ten Thousand Randomly Assorted Digits

	00–04	05–09	10–14	15–19	20–24	25–29	30–34	35–39	40–44	45–49
00	54463	22662	65905	70639	79365	67382	29085	69831	47058	08186
01	15389	85205	18850	39226	42249	90669	96325	23248	60933	26927
02	85941	00756	82414	02015	13858	78030	16269	65978	01385	15345
03	61149	69440	11286	88218	58925	03638	52862	62733	33451	77455
04	05219	81619	10651	67079	92511	59888	84502	72095	83463	75577
05	41417	98326	87719	92294	46614	50948	64886	20002	97365	30976
06	28357	94070	20652	35774	16249	75019	21145	05217	47286	76305
07	17783	00015	10806	83091	91530	36466	39981	62481	49177	75779
08	40950	84820	29881	85966	62800	70326	84740	62660	77379	90279
09	82995	64157	66164	41180	10089	41757	78258	96488	88629	37231
10	96754	17676	55659	44105	47361	34833	86679	23930	53249	27083
11	34357	88040	53364	71726	45690	66334	60332	22554	90600	71113
12	06318	37403	49927	57715	50423	67372	63116	48888	21505	80182
13	62111	52820	07243	79931	89292	84767	85693	73947	22278	11551
14	47534	09243	67879	00544	23410	12740	02540	54440	32949	13491
15	98614	75993	84460	62846	59844	14922	48730	73443	48167	34770
16	24856	03648	44898	09351	98795	18644	39765	71058	90368	44104
17	96887	12479	80621	66223	86085	78285	02432	53342	42846	94771
18	90801	21472	42815	77408	37390	76766	52615	32141	30268	18106
19	55165	77312	83666	36028	28420	70219	81369	41943	47366	41067

20	75884	12952	84318	95108	72305	64620	91318	89872	45375	85436
21	16777	37116	58550	42958	21460	43910	01175	87894	81378	10620
22	46230	43877	80207	88877	89380	32992	91380	03164	98656	59337
23	42902	66892	46134	01432	94710	23474	20423	60137	60609	13119
24	81007	00333	39693	28039	10154	95425	39220	19774	31782	49037
25	68089	01122	51111	72373	06902	74373	96199	97017	41273	21546
26	20411	67081	89950	16944	93054	87687	96693	87236	77054	33848
27	58212	13160	06468	15718	82627	76999	05999	58680	96739	63700
28	70577	42866	24969	61210	76046	67699	42054	12696	93758	03283
29	94522	74358	71659	62038	79643	79169	44741	05437	39038	13163
30	42626	86819	85651	88678	17401	03252	99547	32404	17918	62880
31	16051	33763	57194	16752	54450	19031	58580	47629	54132	60631
32	08244	27647	33851	44705	94211	46716	11738	55784	95374	72655
33	59497	04392	09419	89964	51211	04894	72882	17805	21896	83864
34	97155	13428	40293	09985	58434	01412	69124	82171	59058	82859
35	98409	66162	95763	47420	20792	61527	20441	39435	11859	41567
36	45476	84882	65109	96597	25930	66790	65706	61203	53634	22557
37	89300	69700	50741	30329	11658	23166	05400	66669	48708	03887
38	50051	95137	91631	66315	91428	12275	24816	68091	71710	33258
39	31753	85178	31310	89642	98364	02306	24617	09609	83942	22716

Table 7-1. *(Continued)*

	00–04	05–09	10–14	15–19	20–24	25–29	30–34	35–39	40–44	45–49
40	79152	53829	77250	20190	56535	18760	69942	77448	33278	48805
41	44560	38750	83635	56540	64900	42912	13953	79149	18710	68618
42	68328	83378	63369	71381	39564	05615	42451	64559	97501	65747
43	46939	38689	58625	08342	30459	85863	20781	09284	26333	91777
44	83544	86141	15707	96256	23068	13782	08467	89469	93842	55349
45	91621	00881	04900	54224	46177	55309	17852	27491	89415	23466
46	91896	67126	04151	03795	59077	11848	12630	98375	52068	60142
47	55751	62515	21108	80830	02263	29303	37204	96926	30506	09808
48	85156	87689	95493	88842	00664	55017	55539	17771	69448	87530
49	07521	56898	12236	60277	39102	62315	12239	07105	11844	01117

01385. Bob J. has number 01 and becomes the second member of the group one. Continue to move across rows until five patients for group one have been selected. The remaining five patients are assigned to group two.

Even in this simple example, it can be seen that several numbers whose values did not fall within our range of 1 to 10 were skipped. Several rows would be needed before the randomization process would be completed. In a larger study with a wider range of numbers, several pages of the random number table may be needed before all subjects could be assigned to study groups.

The same number can appear several times in the table. This might occur for the following reason. Since the number is generated in a random fashion, each number has the chance of appearing once, several times, or not at all. Once a number is used to make a group assignment, its subsequent appearance should be disregarded.

After patients are assigned to study groups, it is useful to validate the effectiveness of the randomization procedure. This can be accomplished in two ways. The two groups can be compared to determine whether certain characteristics of subjects (e.g., race, sex) are equally distributed across groups. Or, if there are characteristics of the subjects known to affect the outcome (e.g., age affecting length of hospitalization), the researcher may want to examine the distribution of these factors for each study group. If these known variables are distributed fairly equally, it can be assumed that other, unknown characteristics have similar distributions. If, however, the distributions of these known factors are skewed, that is, younger patients tend to be assigned to one group, the investigator would want to examine the randomization process before proceeding further. It may be necessary to renew the selection process or to control deliberately for the extraneous factors by matching subjects. Matching will be considered in detail in the discussion of quasi-experimental designs.

The last step in the randomization process is the assignment of study groups to treatment modalities. This represents another level of randomization and an additional attempt is to eliminate bias. In this example, group therapy treatment is designated *heads* and the treatment currently in use on the alcohol unit *tails*. A simple flip of the coin determines if group one is assigned to group therapy or standard treatment. When the researcher has more than two study groups, a coin flip cannot be used to determine their assignment. Once again, the random number table is useful for making group assignment decisions. First, identify a new random starting point and determine new procedures for drawing numbers. Let us say that the researcher wants to compare the effects of three treatments for alocholic patients: the standard treatment used on the unit, group therapy, and individual therapy. The standard treatment receives number one; group therapy, number two; and individual therapy, number three. The new starting number is 94070, and, reading down the columns, the first single digit identified that is either 1, 2, or 3 is 17676. Patient group one is assigned to the standard treatment. Continuing down the columns, we come to 37403. Group three will receive individual therapy. The remaining group of patients will be involved with group therapy.

In summary, randomization is perhaps the most efficient and acceptable method of producing comparable study groups. Its effectiveness in controlling the influence of unwanted variables on an outcome increases as the number of subjects in the study increases. The success of randomization can be validated by examining the distributions of easily discernable characteristics, for example, subjects' race or sex, as well as the distributions of subject characteristics known to affect the outcome of the study for each study group. Researchers are advised to use randomization in their studies whenever possible.

Control by Design

Experimental designs provide evidence for the time ordering of variables by the inclusion of control or comparison groups. By constructing an experimental group and a control group that are roughly equivalent, the researcher can assume that differences observed in an outcome occurred as a result of the intervention or treatment. Since the researcher controls the timing of the intervention, the temporal effects can clearly be distinguished.

Additionally, use of a control group helps rule out other possible causal factors. Recall that in the previous example, the research interest was in testing the hypothesis that group therapy reduces hospitalization for alcoholic patients. Sometimes clinicians, in their enthusiasm to demonstrate the effectiveness of a particular treatment, will use a one-shot case-study design. A single group (a group of alcoholic patients) receives an intervention (group therapy), and then some outcome (length of hospitalization) is evaluated:

$$X \longrightarrow 0$$

where X is the treated group and 0 is the outcome. Any observed change in the outcome is presumed to be the result of the treatment. It is difficult to attribute a reduction in hospital stay to group therapy without some standard of comparison. As noted previously, several competing explanations can be offered to explain shorter hospitalization. Characteristics of the subjects, such as age, may account for these findings. Reduced hospitalization may have occurred by chance and therefore be totally unrelated to the use of group therapy. Events in the alcohol unit other than the patients' exposure to group therapy may have contributed to a change in hospitalization patterns. Campbell and Stanley (1963) refer to these alternative explanations as *rival hypotheses* and view them as threats to the internal validity of a study.

THREATS TO INTERNAL VALIDITY

Internal validity is the degree to which changes in an outcome or dependent variable are directly attributable to the treatment or intervention. The more the observed changes in an outcome can plausibly be related to factors other than the treatment, the less confidence the researcher has in inferring causality. Threats to internal validity are discussed individually in the following paragraphs.

History

History refers to the occurrence of events in addition to the treatment that can affect the outcome. The influence of history becomes more problematic the longer the time interval between one observation and another. For example, at the same time group therapy is introduced on the alochol unit, a new medication is administered to the patients that relieves many of the side effects of detoxification. Shorter hospitalization may result from the introduction of this medication as well as from the use of group therapy.

True experimental designs control for history threats to internal validity by use of at least one comparison or control group. With two groups, it can be assumed that external factors, like a new medication, are as likely to effect one group as the other. A control group is similar to the treatment group in every respect except in its exposure to the treatment or intervention. The responses of the control group serve as the basis of comparison with the performance of those subjects who receive the treatment.

Maturation

In conducting nursing research, a person must be particularly sensitive to maturational threats to internal validity. Differences in an outcome that can be attributed to biological changes, for example, aging, or fatigue in the subject occurring over time, are maturational effects. As another example, any observed changes in the size of decubitus ulcers for a paraplegic patient may have little to do with the kind of nursing care the patient received and more to do with this patient's healing processes. Maturational effects are problematic only in studies lacking a control group.

Selection Bias

When a researcher is not able to assign randomly subjects to treatment and control groups, selection biases may be present. Selection bias suggests that observed differences in an outcome are a function of differential recruitment into experimental and control groups. Pretest data can be used to judge the initial comparability of the two study groups; but unless random assignment is used, the researcher runs the risk that subtle pretreatment differences existed.

Testing

Testing effects are simply the influence of taking a pretest on the outcome. Let us say that a group of emergency room nurses is given a questionnaire concerning their attitudes toward rape victims. Several sensitivity training sessions designed to acquaint nurses with the physiological and psychological trauma experienced by rape victims are offered. At the end of the sensitivity training sessions, the same attitudinal questionnaire is administered to see if the training has altered the nurses' perceptions of rape victims. In this example, the influence of the training sessions on nurses' attitudes and changes in attitudes that may have resulted from exposure to the pretest could not be distinguished. The initial administration of the questionnaire may have sensitized the nurses to the topic of rape and thus produced changes in their attitudes toward victims. As with history and maturation threats, testing effects can be reduced by using control groups. In this example, a researcher might want to use two control groups; one control group would receive the pre- and posttests but no sensitivity training, and another group designed to control for testing effects would receive only the posttest.

Mortality

Mortality includes differences in outcome that can be attributed to differential dropout of subjects from experimental and control groups.

Problems of mortality or attrition tend to increase as the length of a study increases. Using the previous example, emergency room nurses are randomly assigned to a control and an experimental study group. Both groups are initially surveyed regarding their attitudes about rape victims. The experimental group receives the sensitivity training sessions, after which both groups are resurveyed. In the second survey, less than one-half of the control subjects respond to the questionnaire while all of the experimental group subjects respond. The two groups can no longer be considered equivalent, since over one-half of the control nurses selected themselves out of the study. It is not known how those who dropped out might have answered the second survey. They may have had the most negative attitudes toward rape victims and therefore were reluctant to complete the posttest questionnaire. It is known that any observed differences in attitudes between control and experimental groups can be attributed to the unrepresentative nature of the control group as well as to the effects of the sensitivity training.

Instrumentation

Instrumentation refers to changes in the measuring tools over time which may account for an observed difference in pretest–posttest scores. Although instrumentation effects are most often associated with machines, such as the loss of elasticity in a blood pressure cuff, these effects should be considered when the data collection source is an interviewer or observer. If an interviewer has become more skillful in gathering information between pre- and post-interviews, differences observed in the scores may reflect changes in the interviewer rather than the effect of the treatment or intervention. Training sessions for interviewers prior to fielding a study can greatly reduce instrumentation bias.

Statistical Regression

Statistical regression to the mean occurs when extreme groups are selected as part of a study population. For example, if a group of intellectually handicapped children were picked for a special education program because of their low achievement scores, it is likely that when they are retested their scores will be higher whether or not they have been exposed to a special education program between the two testing periods. Campbell and Stanley (1963) note that these changes in scores are related to measurement errors. The more deviant the score, the greater the measurement error and the more likely the score is to change at the next observation point. Subjects with very low scores on a pretest move up on a second testing, while those scoring high on the pretest will experience some drop in scores on the posttest. A more detailed discussion of regression to the mean can be found in Campbell and Stanley's book (1963). Statistical regression to the mean can be controlled if individuals with extreme scores on a pretest are randomly assigned to experimental and control groups.

THREATS TO EXTERNAL VALIDITY

The external validity of a study refers to the degree to which findings can be generalized to other populations, settings, or circumstances. For nursing research to be effective, its findings must be applicable for actual nursing practice. Tightly controlled experiments in laboratory settings often exhibit high degrees of internal control, but the artificiality of the research setting greatly limits the usefulness of the findings. The ideal study design is one in which the findings are generalizable and in which appropriate controls for internal validity are present.

Threats to external validity represent ways in which the effects of the causal or treatment factors are limited to a specific set of conditions. Three threats to external validity will be discussed next.

Nonrepresentativeness

When the sample does not adequately reflect the population to which the researcher wants to generalize the findings of a study, the findings are considered nonrepresentative. For example, in the study of the effects of primary nursing on staff nurses' job satisfaction, units at one large teaching hospital were assigned either to primary nursing or team nursing. The generalizability of the findings from this study are limited in two respects: nurses were not randomly assigned to units, and the hospital was not randomly sampled from the entire universe of hospitals. Since much of nursing research is conducted in settings in which complete randomization is often not possible, researchers need to be aware of any characteristics that make the sample nonrepresentative. Replications with other samples, for example, conducting the same study in several other large teaching hospitals, will strengthen the generalizability of the results.

Reactive Effects of Testing

Pretesting may affect study subjects so that their responses to the treatment or intervention are changed, and they are no longer representative of the population. By using control subjects for the pretest, the researcher can determine the extent to which pretesting alters the representativeness of the sample.

Reactive Effects of the Setting

When persons are aware that they are participants in a study, findings may be subject to the so-called *Hawthorne effect.* This term is derived from studies conducted at the Hawthorne plant of the Western Electric Company, in which changes in worker productivity were largely due to the workers' knowledge of being in a research study rather than to the actual experimental manipulations, changes in lighting and working hours. Changes in study participants' responses that are a direct result of knowledge of being included in a study are particularly troublesome in nursing research, since the Hawthorne effect can take place at a variety of levels: hospital administrators, nursing staff, and patients. Double-blind studies, in which neither the study subject nor the person who administers the treatment knows who is in the control group and who is in the experimental group, help to reduce this particular threat to external validity.

True experimental designs provide the researcher with the strongest evidence needed to rule out or to infer a causal relationship. Experimental manipulations of the independent or treatment factor meet the requirement of concomitant variation. Use of a control group supplies temporal evidence for a causal relationship as well as assistance in ruling out other competing explanations for the observed relationship. Randomization helps eliminate competing explanations by creating equivalent study groups in which the distributions of known and unknown variables are presumed to be similar. Threats to the internal validity of a study are minimized largely through the use of randomization and control groups.

COMMON EXPERIMENTAL DESIGNS USED IN NURSING RESEARCH

Numerous designs are available for experimental research. Only a few that are commonly used by nurse researchers will be described.

Pretest–Posttest Control Design

The pretest–posttest control design is perhaps the best known and most frequently employed experimental design. It meets the criteria for inferring causality with the minimum number of subjects. A schematic representation of this design is as follows:

R	O_1	X	O_2	(experimental group)
R	O_1		O_2	(control group)

where R represents random assignment of subjects to experimental and control groups, O_1 represents the pretest measurement. X represents the treatment or intervention, and O_2 represents the posttest measurement.*

Suppose that an investigator wants to evaluate the effectiveness of a particular method of teaching adolescents about venereal disease. First a population of adolescents, for example, the adolescent out-patient department of a large metropolitan hospital, is identified. Then adolescents are randomly assigned to treatment and control groups. Each group is pretested to determine its level of knowledge about venereal diseases and their prevention, detection, and treatment. A mean pretest score is computed for each group. Next, the experimental or treatment group is shown a 30 minute film detailing the steps an adolescent should take if it is suspected that he or she has contracted a venereal disease. Both groups are subsequently posttested. A score reflecting the average change in each group's level of knowledge about venereal diseases is computed by subtracting its mean pretest score from its mean posttest score ($O_2 - O_1$). Using an appropriate statistical technique, difference scores for the experimental group are compared with the difference scores for the control group to determine whether seeing a movie on venereal diseases significantly increases adolescents' level of knowledge about the diseases.

This study design provides controls for internal validity. History, maturational, and testing effects should be comparable for experimental and control groups. Selection biases are eliminated by randomization. Use of a self-administered questionnaire helps to reduce instrumentation effects. Regression to the mean can be controlled if subjects whose scores on the pretest are either extremely high or low are randomly assigned to experimental and control groups prior to administration of the treatment. In this way, changes in scores due to regression will occur equally for both groups. Attrition or mortality can be evaluated by comparing the characteristics of those subjects who took both the pre- and posttest with those who took only the pretest.

*Campbell, D.T., Stanley, J.C. *Experimental and Quasi-Experimental Designs for Research.* Chicago: Rand McNally & Company. Copyright 1963. American Educational Research Association, Washington, D.C.

The pretest–posttest design is easily extended to include several variations of the independent variable. For example, in evaluating two teaching methods for venereal diseases, the research design would resemble the following:

R	O_1	X_1	O_2	(method 1)
R	O_1	X_2	O_2	(method 2)
R	O_1		O_2	(control)

In this case, several comparisons are possible. The relative influence of each teaching method on the outcome can be assessed, or the two teaching methods can be compared. The differential effects of the two teaching methods can be determined without a control group; however, a control group allows the researcher to draw more powerful conclusions. (For another nursing example of the extended pretest–posttest design, see Tamez, Moore, and Brown, 1978).

Posttest Control Design

If it is possible to randomize subjects to experimental and control groups, pretesting is not always necessary. If the researcher can establish, with reasonable validity, pretreatment equality between experimental and control groups, then the posttest only design is a simpler, easier way of determining treatment effects. This is the design of choice for those situations in which a pretest is unavailable or when taking a pretest is likely to effect the treatment itself. The design is as follows:

R	X	O_2	(experimental group)
R		O_2	(control group)

In this example, adolescents would be randomly assigned to the experimental and control groups. The experimental group would see a movie on venereal diseases, and then both groups would be tested regarding their knowledge of venereal diseases. With a posttest only design, the pretreatment knowledge levels for the two groups cannot be determined. Suppose the control group had more knowledge about venereal disease than the experimental group prior to the movie intervention. The movie might increase the knowledge of the experimental group, since this group had less knowledge about venereal diseases to begin with, and a comparison of the two groups on a posttest would be likely to yield nonsignificant findings. Similarly, if the control group had less knowledge initially, differences between control and experimental groups on the posttest might be artificially inflated. If randomization is adequate, these initial differences in the two study groups will occur by chance in only 5% of the experiments. Researchers who are unwilling to risk a one in twenty chance that their control and experimental groups are not equivalent will want to pretest.

The Solomon Four-Group Design

The Solomon four-group design represents the most rigorous of all commonly used experimental designs. Here, controls are present for testing effects as well as for treatment effects. Subjects are randomly assigned to one of four groups: an experimental group and three control groups. The design is diagramed

R	O_1	X	O_2	(experimental)
R	O_1		O_2	(control for treatment)
R		X	O_2	(control for pretest)
R			O_2	(control for pretest and treatment)

In this design, two groups receive the treatment *(X)* but only one is pretested (O_1). Similarly, two groups act as controls with only one being pretested. Thus, the interaction effect of the pretest and treatment can be systematically assessed.

Although this design combines the virtues of the pretest–posttest and posttest only designs, it has two major weaknesses. From a practical perspective, it is often difficult to find enough subjects to create four comparable groups. From a statistical viewpoint, analysis of findings is complicated since there are four groups but only three complete sets of measures (pretest, treatment, posttest). While comparisons can be made between subgroups, for example, pretest versus no pretest, difficulties arise when the researcher wants to use some overall statistical procedure that can make use of all sets of observations.

The Solomon four-group design is useful when there is a large pool of potential subjects, when findings from previous experiments with simpler designs suggest hypotheses that demand greater rigor and control, and when the major focus of the analysis is to make subgroup comparisons.

Factorial Designs

Traditional experimental designs are constructed so that a single factor *X* varies while all other conditions are held constant. In a sense, this is an artificial situation, since in the real world relationships between phenomena are far more complex. Factorial designs allow the researcher to analyze the effects of two or more factors simultaneously. Additionally, factorial designs provide information on whether factors interact to produce differences in the outcome that would not occur if each factor were considered separately.

Factorial designs, therefore, have several advantages over traditional experimental designs. They allow the researcher to test several hypotheses at one time rather than having to conduct a series of single-factor experiments. They permit the simultaneous testing of interaction effects.

An example of a simple factorial design is the 2 × 2 design in which the effects of two treatments are varied in two ways. For example, let us say that the researcher wants to evaluate two teaching methods for venereal disease and two lengths of time for the teaching period. The 2 × 2 design would resemble that shown in Figure 7-1, where X_1 represents the two teaching methods and X_2 represents the two lengths of class time. Adolescents are randomly assigned to each of the four groups. Group A receives a 60-minute discussion on venereal disease, Group B's discussion is limited to 30 minutes, Group C receives a lecture and sees a movie for 60 minutes, and Group D sees the same movie and lecture for 30 minutes.

Following administration of these two teaching methods, all adolescents are evaluated to determine their level of knowledge about venereal diseases. Mean scores are computed for each group as well as mean scores for pairs of groups that experienced the same teaching methods (e.g., A + B) and pairs that experienced the same length of class time (e.g., A + C).

From these data, several questions can be answered: What is the main

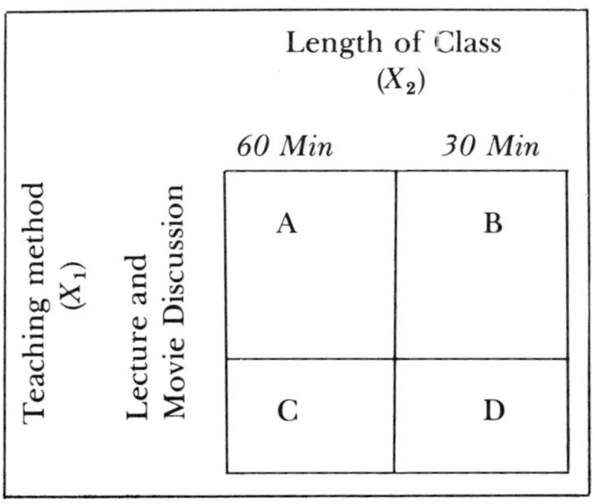

Figure 7-1. Factorial experimental 2×2 design.

effect of the teaching method on adolescents' knowledge of venereal diseases? What is the main effect of length of instruction? Is there an interaction effect of type of teaching method and length of class on knowledge about venereal diseases? If the effect of the method of teaching on adolescents' level of knowledge varies with the length of the class period, there is an interaction effect present.

Factorial designs are an effective and efficient way to test for interactions and to test multiple hypotheses in a single study. This simple 2 × 2 design is easily extended to permit evaluation of several teaching methods at multiple levels (e.g., 2 × 3, 2 × 2 × 2). Multivariate statistical techniques are available to analyze findings from more complex factorial designs (see Cochran and Cox, 1957).

QUASI-EXPERIMENTAL DESIGNS

Nurse researchers frequently find themselves in situations in which they lack complete control over those properties that characterize true experiments: randomization, experimental manipulation, and control by comparison. These researchers might not have the opportunity to randomly assign subjects to experimental and control groups. They may be required to give the treatment to all subjects and thus lack a control or comparison group. This situation often occurs in clinical settings in which it is impossible to offer a treatment to one group of patients and withold the treatment from another group. Campbell and Stanley (1963, 1966) have developed several research designs applicable to situations in which the researcher is unable to make random assignments or use control groups but can manipulate a treatment or intervention factor. These designs are called *quasi-experimental,* since they share some but not all of the characteristics of true experiments. An example of a quasi-experimental design can be found in Vincent and Price (1977).

The Nonequivalent Control Group Design

The nonequivalent control group design differs from the pretest–posttest control groups experimental design in that the researcher is unable to make random assignments of subjects to treatment and control groups. Suppose a researcher wanted to evaluate the impact of primary nursing on nurses' job satisfaction. The researcher is unable randomly to assign nurses to primary units and team nursing units, since the nursing units are already constituted groups. Therefore, units are randomized to primary (experimental) or team (control) methods of nursing care. The design would resemble the following:

R	O_1	X	O_2	(experimental group)
R	O_1		O_2	(control group)

Nurses' perceived job satisfaction would be measured at O_1. One unit would then use primary nursing as a method of nursing care organization *(X)*, and the nurses' job satisfaction for each unit would be reassessed at some later point in time (O_2).

The effectiveness of this design is dependent on how strong a case can be made for the comparability of the two groups before the implementation of primary nursing. If the nurses had responded similarly on the pretest (O_1), then it may be assumed that any observed differences in posttest job satisfaction (O_2) were attributable to the method of nursing care organization. If, however, the perceived level of job satisfaction for the two groups was very different initially, any observed differences in job satisfaction following the implementation of primary nursing could not be easily interpreted.

Matching

Since quasi-experimental designs lack some of the controls of true experiments, the researcher often attempts to build in additional controls as a way of compensating for the lack of randomization. One such control is matching. Matching is a procedure for creating equivalent study groups in the absence of randomization. It necessitates prior knowledge of subject characteristics. The researcher begins with subjects who are receiving the treatment or intervention and then attempts to create a control group by matching each individual in the treatment group with another individual in the general population on characteristics that presumably have an effect on the outcome under study. Matching is an ex post facto strategy for reducing the number of competing or rival hypotheses for an observed relationship.

While matching does increase the strength of quasi-experimental designs, it is not without pitfalls. Effective matching is dependent on the researcher's prior knowledge about certain characteristics of subjects and the relationship of these characteristics to some outcome. Additionally, it is difficult to use matching when the researcher wants to control for more than two or three variables. Suppose, in the investigation of the impact of primary nursing on nurses' job satisfaction, the researcher wanted to control for age, race, and educational background of nurses. For every nurse on a primary nursing unit, it would be necessary to identify a nurse with the same age, race, and educational training who uses another form of nursing care organization. Often it is impossible to find identical matches, therefore it is necessary to match individuals having approximately the same characteristics to serve in the control group (e.g., a subject aged 30 matched with a subject aged 28). Matching represents one strategy for introducing control into quasi-experimental designs. Also, there are statistical procedures, such as analysis of covariance, which will adjust for initial differences in the study groups in the analysis of the data.

Time Series Designs

Time series designs are based on the premise that information can be collected on a group of subjects over a period of time and that the effects of a treatment or intervention over the same time period can also be assessed. The design is diagramed as follows:

Week → 1 → 2 → 3 → 4 → 5 → 6 → 7 → 8

O_1 O_2 O_3 O_4 X O_5 O_6 O_7 O_8

Pretreatment Posttreatment

where $O_1 \rightarrow O_4$ represent observations on the outcome taken preceding the treatment, and $O_5 \rightarrow O_8$ represent observations following the implementation of the treatment. Measurements $O_1 \rightarrow O_4$ are treated as pretest data, and $O_5 \rightarrow O_8$ serve as posttest data. The effect of X is therefore assumed to be reflected in the difference between pretest and posttest observations.

Using the primary nursing example, let us say that observations O_1 through O_4 represent measurements of nurses' job satisfaction taken after primary nursing has been implemented. Figure 7-2 suggests three possible hypothetical outcome patterns for this particular time series design, where A, B, and C represent nursing units, X represents the introduction of primary nursing, and black dots represent mean job satisfaction scores for nurses on each unit at eight different observation points.

One might infer from these patterns that the introduction of primary nursing has an effect on the average levels of nurses' job satisfaction in units A and B but not in unit C. The outcome pattern for unit C indicates that factors other than primary nursing have an impact on nurses' job satisfaction. The effectiveness of a time series design is

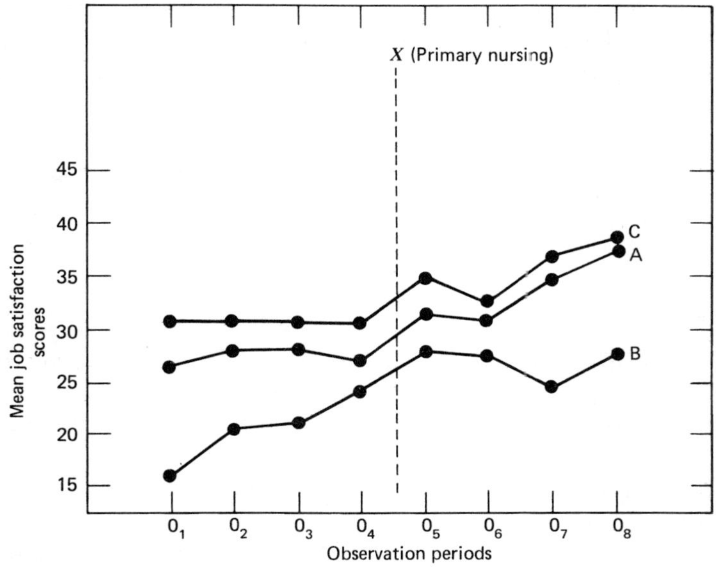

Figure 7-2. Three outcome patterns in a time series experimental design.

dependent on the number of observations and the interval of time between each observation. This design is most appropriate in settings where measurements are routinely gathered at specific time intervals (e.g., vital statistics) or when the researcher knows the rate of change of variables of interest or wishes to learn a rate of change. For example, if the researcher wishes to study the relationship between a hospital staff nurse's perceived job satisfaction and subsequent turnover, it is important that the researcher know something about nursing turnover rates. Suppose turnover has a seasonal pattern, with the greatest proportion of newly hired nurses arriving in September and October and the turnover rates peaking in the late spring and early summer months. Unless the researcher selects a measurement interval that taps the nurse's perceived job satisfaction just prior to the peak resignation months, invalid conclusions may be drawn from the data. Time series study designs presume, therefore, that previous research has not only identified appropriate variables but has determined their rate of change and the frequency of occurrence of other events between measurements.

Quasi-experimental research lacks the controls present in true experimental designs that permit causal inferences. Yet, if only true experimental designs were permitted in nursing research, most of the studies would be confined to laboratories and be of little practical use to nurse clinicians. The strength of quasi-experimental research lies in its ability to adapt to a variety of real world settings. This practical aspect makes quasi-experimental designs attractive research alternatives to nurses in clinical areas. It is important that researchers who use quasi-experimental designs are cognizant of their weaknesses and understand how the lack of control affects the interpretation of findings.

SUMMARY

Research designs serve as blueprints for conducting empirical studies. Each design contains a set of rules or requirements that provide guidance in deciding what, where, when, and how to test relationships between observed phenomena. The decision to select one research design over another is dependent on 1) the purpose of the study and 2) the nature of the problem.

Research studies vary depending on their level. Exploratory or formulative studies are useful for concept formation, theory development, and for establishing research priorities in an area of interest. Descriptive studies provide a detailed accounting of a population, event, or situation and are useful in examining relationships between phenomena. The purpose of experimental research is to test cause–effect relationships. Three criteria were identified for inferring causality: concomitant variation, temporal ordering of variables, and evidence that rules out other possible causal factors. Concomitant variation refers to the extent to which the independent and dependent variables occur together in the hypothesized direction. In an experimental study, the researcher provides evidence for concomitant variation by manipulating the independent variable (treatment or intervention) and then observing the effect of that action on a particular outcome. The second criterion, temporal ordering, is met by including a control group or comparison group whose performance on the outcome serves as a basis for evaluating the performance of the experimental or treatment group. The researcher is able to obtain measures on the outcome for both groups before the treatment and after the treatment. In this way, observed differences in the outcome between control and treatment groups can be attributed to the effect of the treatment. The third criterion for inferring causality, evidence ruling out other competing hypotheses, can be met by use of randomization and control groups. Random assignment procedure gives each subject an equal chance of being assigned to the treatment or control groups, thereby decreasing the possibility that factors other than the treatment are likely to account for observed differences in outcome. Randomization does not always succeed in producing equivalent groups, but it is the most effective technique available for creating comparable groups. Specific competing or rival hypotheses were discussed. These include history, maturation, testing, mortality, instrumental effects, and statistical regression to the mean. These competing hypotheses, often referred to as threats to internal validity of a study, are usually eliminated or their effects are reduced by randomization and the use of control groups. External validity, or the generalizability of study findings, was also discussed.

Two major types of experimental designs were presented: true experiments and quasi-experiments. True experiments and quasi-experiments differ largely on the degree of control the researcher has over the study environment and over extraneous or unwanted variables. True experiments are characterized by randomization, manipulation of the causal factor, and use of control or comparison groups. True experiments provide the strongest evidence for inferring cause-effect relationships and, as such, represent the ideals of scientific inquiry, prediction, and explanation. Quasi-experimental designs involve manipulation of the causal factor but frequently lack randomization and control groups. Other controls, such as matching, can be introduced into quasi-experimental studies as a means of creating comparable study groups. These compensatory mechanisms strengthen quasi-experimental research but are unable completely to remove all competing or rival hypotheses. The major strength of quasi-experimental designs lies in their practicality, feasibility, and applicability to clinical settings.

BIBIOGRAPHY

Campbell, D.T., & Stanley, J. C. *Experimental and Quasi-Experimental Designs for Research.* Chicago: Rand McNally and Company, Copyright 1963, American Educational Research Association, Washington, D.C.

Cochran, W. G., & Cox, G. *Experimental Designs,* 2nd Edition. New York: John Wiley & Sons, 1957.

Felton, G. Increasing the quality of nursing care by introducing the concept of primary nursing: A model project. *Nursing Research,* 1975, *24,* pp. 27–32.

Gerber, R. A., and Van Ort, S. R. Topical application of insulin in decubitus ulcers. *Nursing Research,* 1979, *28,* pp. 16–19.

Griggs, B. A systems approach to the development and evaluation of a mini-course for nurses. *Nursing Research,* 1977, *26,* pp. 34–41.

Kerlinger, F. N. *Foundations of Behavioral Research,* 2nd Edition. New York: Holt, Rinehart and Winston, 1973.

Reider, K., and Wood, M. Problem-orientation: An experimental study to test its heuristic value. *Nursing Research,* 1978, *27,* pp. 25–29.

Selltiz, C., Wrightsman, L. S., and Cook, S.W. *Research Methods in Social Relations,* 3rd Edition. New York: Holt, Rinehart and Winston, 1976.

Tamez, E., Moore, M., and Brown, P. Relaxation training as a nursing intervention versus Pro Re Nata medication. *Nursing Research,* 1978, *27,* pp. 160–164.

Vincent, P., and Price, J. R. Evaluation of a VNA mental health project. *Nursing Research,* 1977, *26,* pp. 361–367.

8
Aspects of Measurement

Phyllis Giovannetti

Measurement is the basis of all science. Whether one is interested in developing the skills necessary to conduct research or peruse the results, knowledge of the process and problems of measurement is crucial. While the concept of measurement and the issues presented in this chapter are not difficult, obtaining precise measurements can often be a frustrating experience. The more abstract the concept, the more challenging is the process of measurement. It is perhaps for this reason that the contribution of those who have developed precise measurement devices has been highly regarded in the research field.

Chapter 8 first discusses the rules that are needed to assign numbers to the events under study. The rules are important, for they have a direct bearing on the quality of the measurement procedure. The rules also define the measurement scale or level of measurement that may be applied. Four levels of measurement—nominal, ordinal, interval, and ratio—are presented, along with the appropriate inferences that can be made with each level. The chapter discusses in detail potential measurement errors in terms of random and constant errors. If they occur, these errors can affect the results of measurement by masking the true differences in the objects being measured.

Finally, the chapter includes a detailed discussion of reliability and validity as they relate to the subject of measurement. Both concepts are important because the value of a measurement procedure depends upon the extent to which it possesses the attributes of reliability and validity.

THE NATURE OF MEASUREMENT

Measurement refers to the assignment of numbers to objects or events, or properties of objects or events, according to a set of rules. A *numeral* is a symbol such as 1, 2, 3, . . . or I, II, III, . . . and has no quantitative meaning unless we give it such a meaning. For example, a technician taking blood samples from a patient might choose to label them 1, 2, 3, and so forth, in which case the numbers would be used as labels. It would not make any sense to add the first two specimens and equate that with the 3 relating to the third specimen. Once assignment of a quantitative meaning is given to a numeral, it becomes a *number*.

Rules represent the instructions, guides, or methods that are used to assign the numerals or numbers to data or events under study. For example, a measurement rule might say: "Assign the numerals I, II, III to patients on a nursing unit, according to their mobility status. If the patient can ambulate by himself, let the numeral be I. If the patient requires some assistance, let the numeral be II. If the patient requires total assistance, let the numeral be III." Another rule might be: "If the person is a female, assign her a 1. If a person is a male, assign him a 0." As another example, suppose there are five nursing students and the instructor wishes to assign a rank of 1 to the student with the greatest nursing ability, a rank of 2 to the student with the next greatest nursing ability, and so on to the rank of 5, which would be assigned to the student with the least nursing ability.

Obviously, for all three examples, a prior set of rules defining sex, ambulation, and nursing ability would be needed. The measurement of sex is not likely to be too difficult, as several simple and clear criteria can be used to determine whether one is male or female. Other human characteristics, such as height and weight, are also easily measured. Ambulation may be a little more difficult; but again, simple and clear criteria, that is good rules, can be established. Many human characteristics, however, including our example of nursing ability, can be very difficult to measure, because clear and concise rules are not readily identifiable.

Rules are the most significant component of the measurement procedure, because they can determine the quality of measurement. Poor rules can render measurement meaningless, because they do not tie the measurement procedure to reality. To use a simple example, if the rule used to assign sex suggested that short-haired persons were male and long-haired persons were female, one would have little confidence in the outcome of the measurement.

Frequently, researchers are interested in measuring properties or characteristics of objects, or indicators of properties, rather than the objects themselves. Properties such as satisfaction and motivation cannot be directly observed. They must be inferred from the observation of some presumed indicators of the properties. If a patient achieves a certain score on a satisfaction questionnaire, we can infer something about that patient's level of satisfaction. In other words, some identifiable behavior is an indicator of an underlying property. The process of measuring indicators of properties is identical with the process for measuring directly observable properties. The rules, however, are much more difficult to formulate for measuring indicators of properties, and the researcher must rely to some degree on inference.

LEVELS OF MEASUREMENT

Rules are also important because they define the kind of measurement scale or level of measurement that is to be applied to the observations. Four distinct levels of measurement are commonly referred to: nominal, ordinal, interval, and ratio. They concern the different uses made of the numerals or numbers that are assigned to objects or events during the process of measurement. The operations that can be performed on a given set of numbers, and thus the inferences that can be made about the data, are dependent on the level of measurement attained.

Nominal Level

The weakest level of measurement is the nominal level. Numbers, symbols, or other labels are used only to classify the objects measured. For instance, the numerals 1 and 2 could be used to classify a group of students into males and females, with 1 representing females and 2 representing males. Or a group of patients could be classified as medical, surgical, or obstetrical, depending upon the clinical specialty to which they are assigned. The level of measurement would remain unchanged if the researcher preferred to classify the patients as 1, 2, 3, with 1 representing medical, 2 surgical, and 3 obstetrical.

The conclusions one can draw from nominal data are limited; hence, the notion of the "weakest level of measurement." Only one inference can be made. That is, for the preceding examples, the two groups of students are of different sexes, or the patients are different with respect to clinical specialty. Only nonquantitative statistical procedures are appropriate for nominal data. One can logically discuss the number (frequency) of male and female students or the percentage of students who are male and female, but it makes little sense to speak of the range, mean, or standard deviation of the sexes. For the patients classified according to clinical specialty, the same statistics apply; although because there are more than two categories, the mode is also appropriately used. Thus, for nominal scales, there is little quantitative aspect to the data, and they can be subject to few computational processes.

Ordinal Level

There are other properties that not only can be classified but also identified as having some relationship to each other. Patient classification systems in which patients are grouped into categories according to their requirements for nursing care are presented as a good example. Category I represents those patients requiring a minimal amount of care; Category II, an average amount of care; and Category III, an above-average amount of care. The data are considered ordinal, not only because the patients' requirements for care are different, but also because comparative judgments can be made in terms of more or less care. Thus, one can draw two sets of conclusions: 1) The patients in each category of care are different; and 2) patients in Category III require more care than those in Categories I and II, and patients in Category II require more care than those in Category I.

Measurement at the ordinal level is also commonly found in studies of attitudes. For example, five respondents might be asked to mark the number representing their degree of agreement or disagreement with a set of statements relating to a proposed hospital policy change. Assume a researcher uses 20 statements, each of which has four alternative answers, with 1 standing for "totally disagree," 2 for "partially disagree," 3 for "partially agree," and 4 for "totally agree." A total score of 80, representing a score of 4 on each of the 20 items, would be the highest score achievable. Assuming that all respondents answered all questions, a respondent with a score of 80 might be regarded as having the most positive attitude toward the proposed policy and could be ranked first. Table 8–1 displays hypothetical scores and ranks of five respondents.

Table 8-1. Ranking Respondents by Their Attitude Toward a Policy Change

Respondent	*Score*	*Rank*
1	40	4th
2	20	5th
3	52	3rd
4	80	1st
5	76	2nd

The next highest score (76) goes to respondent 5, who would then be ranked second. Examination of the table reveals that respondent 4 has the most favorable attitude toward the policy, while respondent 2 has the least favorable attitude toward the policy. It is important to note that the ordinal values, 1st, 2nd, 3rd, represent rank orders and nothing more. The numbers do not indicate that the intervals between the numbers are equal, nor do they indicate absolute quantities. All that can be said is that the respondents have different ranks and that rank 1 exceeds ranks 2 to 5.

Interval Level

At the interval level of measurement, units of measurement are used. These units refer to the distance between each of the objects being measured. In this instance, a real number is assigned to the object under measurement. Fahrenheit temperature is a good example of an interval scale. If the researcher were to measure the temperatures of two patients and find one to be 102°F and the other 98.6°F, it would be correct to draw three conclusions: 1) the two patients have different temperatures; 2) one patient's temperature is higher than the other; 3) one patient's temperature is 3.4°F higher than the other. Many educational and psychological tests make use of interval scales with the application of + (more than) or − (less than) expressions.

The nature of the interval level of measurement provides the researcher with greater scope in analysis and thus in the inferences that can be drawn. As previously noted with interval data one can determine the exact and equal distance between the objects measured. Whereas use of such measures as the mean and standard deviation were inappropriate for nominal and ordinal data, they are quite meaningful for interval data.

Ratio Level

The highest level of measurement is referred to as the ratio level. Properties that have natural zero points can be measured on the ratio scale. A natural, or true, zero point is defined as the total absence of the quantity being measured. It is not the same as the zero that exists in many ordinal and interval scales, such as the zero in the Fahrenheit scale. The true zero in the Fahrenheit scale is actually −460°, although the measure of thermal activity is begun at an artificial zero placed in the upper reaches of the scale.

All arithmetic operations, including multiplication and division, can be applied to variables measured at the ratio level. As the name implies, the ratio concept can be used in describing the data. If the researcher were to determine that one person was 60 years of age and another person 30 years of age, four conclusions could be drawn from the determination: 1) the two persons have different ages; 2) one person is older than the other; 3) one person is 30 years older than the other; and 4) one person is two times as old as the other. It should thus be apparent that variables measured at the ratio level of measurement can also be measured at the interval, ordinal, and nominal levels. The converse is not true, however. Variables measured at the lower levels cannot be measured at the higher levels. Interval and ratio measures are common in the physical sciences for a wide variety of variables. In the social sciences, attaining the higher levels of a measurement is much more difficult.

In summary, the process of assigning a value or score to observations constitutes the process of measurement. The rules for defining the assignment of an appropriate value determine the level or scale of measurement. The four levels discussed differ in relation to the classifying, ordering, and distancing properties inherent in the measurement rules. The specific level of measurement achieved or selected determines which statistical techniques can be used and, thus, the inferences that can be made. As will become clear after reading Part 4 of this book, each statistical technique is appropriate for specific levels of measurement.

MEASUREMENT ERRORS

During the process of measurement, many factors may affect both the characteristics being measured and the process of measurement itself. The importance of research designs in attempting to control for the more important of these variables is discussed in Chapter 7. Nevertheless, the dynamic nature of measurement and the complex environment in which it takes place limit the researcher's attempts at control. As a result, the variations among the results of measurement may reflect not only the characteristics of interest but also other known and unknown factors. True differences between the objects in the characteristic being measured may account for some of the variations. In the ideal measuring situation, all of the differences between the objects in the characteristic being measured would be true differences. For example, if a questionnaire is supposed to measure patient satisfaction with nursing care, all the differences in scores among the sample would reflect the patients' differing levels of satisfaction. No differences would reflect chance variation, the effects of other characteristics or attitudes of the patients, or features of the questionnaire itself. The fact is, however, that other sources of differences do exist and enter into the results of measurement. These represent *errors of measurement.*

Errors of measurement are customarily classified into two groups: *unsystematic,* or *random,* errors, and *systematic,* or *constant,* errors. The goal in measurement is to reduce the effects of error so that the instrument approaches as nearly as possible the perfect instrument to be used in the ideal measurement situation.

Random errors are introduced into measurement by factors that are likely to vary from one act of measurement to the next. These include transient aspects of the person, of the situation of measurement, or of the measurement procedures. The following is a list of factors that may be responsible for producing unsystematic, or random, errors. It is important to recognize these factors as probable sources of differences in measurement and to attempt to reduce their impact on measurement instruments and procedures.

1. *Factors relating to the respondent or subject.* Various personal factors, such as mood, motivation, health, attention span, state of fatigue, and so on, may vary within a short period of time and affect the subject's response. Selltiz, Wrightsman, and Cook (1976) define these as "transient personal factors" and suggest that their influence may depend on the way the respondent defines the situation of measurement. For example, asking a group of busy people to complete a lengthy questionnaire may result in their rushing through what seems to them to be a trivial and irrelevant exercise. Generally, the effect of these transient personal factors can be reduced by establishing appropriate conditions of motivation and rapport prior to measurement.

2. *Factors relating to the observer.* Transient personal factors may also affect the way in which an observer makes the measurements. The observer may become tired or bored and careless in the recording of observations. Inadequate and nonuniform methods of administering an instrument may also contribute to variations in the scores. In the case of an interview, the interviewer may omit questions, change the wording, or revise the order in such a way as to make one interview incomparable with another. The subject's response or the observer's interpretation of the subject's response may be affected. How the observer or interviewer defines the situation of measurement and, in some cases, how central the topic is to the observer may also affect the outcome. Selecting a nurse, whose outspoken views on the poor quality of nursing care are wellknown, to participate in a nursing audit may result in observations that primarily reflect the nurse's bias. Thus, both the consistency with

which an observer or coder rates the responses of various individuals and the consistency of ratings from one observer or coder to another may be affected. These effects can be lessened by thoughtful selection and appropriate training, motivation, and pilot testing as well as good supervision of data collectors before actual measurement.

3. *Factors relating to the situation of measurement.* The conditions or situations under which measurement is taken may cause changes in the results that do not reflect true variations. For instance, an interview with a patient about the quality of nursing care may be greatly affected if the interviewer is a nurse known to the patient, if the patient's family is present, or if anonymity is not assured. These factors represent constant sources of error.

The situations of measurement may also be differently affected by various noise distractions, an atmosphere of playfulness or seriousness, or the lack of rapport. The situation of measurement may vary from person to person or from one set of measurements to another, resulting in considerable variation in scores apart from the true differences among people with respect to the attribute being measured. Further, attention should be given to the situation of measurement for such things as time of day, external conditions, and general atmosphere.

4. *Factors relating to the instrument.* Characteristics of the instrument itself may affect responses. Lack of clarity of the instrument or the instructions, the use of emotionally colored words, or the use of words with ambiguous meanings may cause variations in response that reflect differences in interpretation rather than differences in the characteristic being measured. For instance, a quality audit may have as one of the questions "Are allergies recorded?" While one auditor may record "yes" because the patient did not have any allergies, another may record "no" because no allergies were recorded.

Mechanical factors associated with the instrument may also be the cause of variations. A questionnaire that is neatly spaced and typed may affect responses differently than one that is carelessly prepared and printed. Pretesting instruments on a subsample of respondents as similar as possible to the target population is critical to the identification of some of these problems.

Variation in responses may also be affected by the items contained in the instrument. Most measuring instruments necessarily contain only a portion of all the possible questions, statements, or observations relevant to the characteristic being measured. Thus, a quality of care instrument contains only a few items from the total universe of items that might have been included to describe quality care. Variations in quality measured by different instruments will be dependent, in part, on the nature of the sample of items included in the instruments. Even within the same instrument, variations may occur because different aspects of quality may be more important for different types of patients.

5. *Factors relating to processing and analysis. Random,* or unsystematic, errors may occur in the coding, scoring, tabulation, machine analysis, and statistical computations associated with the measuring instrument. Errors of this kind, however, are easier to avoid or control. As a matter of routine, systematic checks should be made at each stage of the processing and analysis to identify and correct errors.

The preceding list of factors represents some of the principal sources of errors known as random, or unsystematic, errors. The number and kind of factors of concern to an investigator will depend on the nature of the instrument and how it is to be used. Interviews, questionnaires, objective tests, and evaluative measures all have unique features that render some sources of random error more significant than others. In addition to random errors, it has been noted that measurement can also be affected by *constant,* or systematic, errors.

Constant errors are those that are introduced into measurement by some factor that systematically affects the characteristics being measured or the process of measurement. Stable personal factors such as intelligence, education, social status, information, and personality characteristics of the person can contribute to constant errors. Two such characteristics that, in particular, can affect responses to interviews and questionnaires include the tendency to give a favorable impression of one's self and the tendency to agree (or disagree) with statements regardless of their content. These are frequently referred to as the "social desirability" influence and the "acquiescent response set." For example, if respondents are asked to indicate their agreement or disagreement with statements that are subject to considerations of social desirability, differences in scores may reflect differences in respondents' willingness to admit holding "undesirable" positions as well as differences in the characteristic the instrument is intended to measure. The respondents must be assured that they will not be penalized for their types of answers.

The tendency to agree or disagree with a series of statements regardless of the content may be a stable personality characteristic of some respondents, or it may be characteristic of the measuring instrument. Nevertheless, the potential for systematic errors must be considered, and investigators should make every effort to assure that their measurements are free from these influences.

Factors representing sources of error have a direct effect on the reliability and validity of measuring instruments. Estimates of reliability consider primarily the effects of random errors. As suggested by Suchman (1967), reliability can best be controlled by careful attention to those factors that permit large chance errors to enter into measurement. Estimates of validity are concerned with both constant and random errors.

RELIABILITY

Reliability refers to the concept of consistency or repeatability. When referring to the reliability of an instrument or measurement procedure, we mean the degree to which the instrument can be depended upon to yield consistent results upon repeated applications. A reliable measure of length, such as a yardstick, can be expected to yield the same measurement of a table each time the table is measured. If it does not, then the yardstick lacks perfect reliability and contains measurement error. A measure of "satisfaction with pay level" would be unreliable if it measured the same person as "highly satisfied" on one occasion and "totally dissatisfied" on a second occasion when both measurements were taken under similar circumstances; that is, the person had not received a pay raise.

As previously noted, any measure can be thought of as containing two components: 1) a true score, which is the real value of the variable of interest, and 2) measurement error. An unreliable measure contains a large component of measurement error and thus does not provide an accurate measure. A reliable measure, on the other hand, contains little or no measurement error and thus can provide an accurate measure. The concept of true score and measurement error can be conveyed as follows. Suppose there are two thermometers, one that is highly reliable and one that is not reliable. An obtained reading of 98.6° on the first one and 101° on the second, taken simultaneously on both thermometers, might be shown as in Figure 8–1.

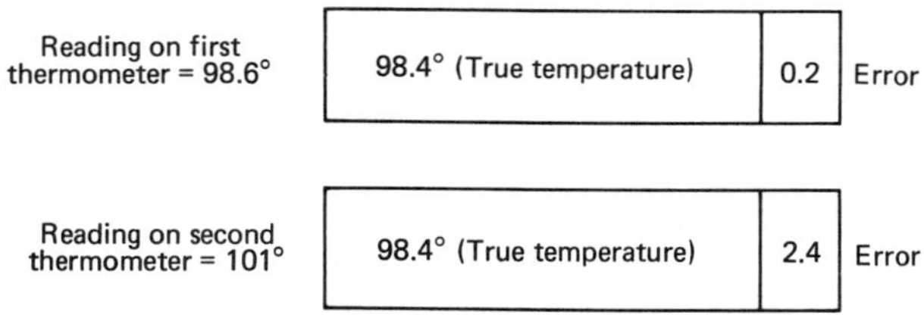

Figure 8-1. Readings on Two Thermometers.

The second thermometer is less reliable than the first because it has greater measurement error. It should be noted that the second thermometer could consistently provide the same invalid reading. It does not yield a consistent or precise measurement of body temperature.

The importance of reliability is obvious. An unreliable measure of a variable, such as satisfaction with pay, would be useless in studying that variable, and an unreliable thermometer would be useless in measuring a patient's body temperature.

Although the concept of reliability as a measure of consistency or repeatability appears to be simple, there are, in fact, several aspects of reliability and a variety of methods appropriate for estimating these different aspects. The three aspects of reliability that are most commonly referred to are measures of *stability, equivalence,* and *homogeneity.*

Before discussing the three aspects of reliability, it is important to note that reliability is frequently defined as a "correlation coefficient." This definition undoubtedly stemmed from the common practice of estimating reliability through correlational statistics. Such a definition, however, is both misleading and inaccurate. Although correlational procedures are appropriate in some instances, they are quite inappropriate in others. This point will be discussed in more detail later in this chapter.

Stability refers to the consistency of measures on repeated applications. In other words, how stable is a person's position on a measure from one administration to another? The most common measure of stability is the procedure known as *test-retest* reliability. A measuring instrument such as a questionnaire, interview, or test is usually administered to the same group of persons at two different times, and the two sets of scores are then compared. When the measuring instrument consists of observations, a number of repeated observations may be made. Several problems are encountered with the test-retest method. First, the fact that a person has once been tested may influence the second measurement. For example respondents to a questionnaire or interview may remember their initial response and attempt to give the same response at the second measurement period. Thus, the results might appear to be more consistent than they actually are. Second, transient personal factors may become more intense on the second measurement. Respondents may become more anxious, tired, or bored. Third, the initial measure may affect the second measure by stimulating respondents to change their attitude, behavior, or knowledge. For example, asking a nurse about her attitude toward students in a new program may heighten her interest in the students, causing her to discuss and inquire about the program and thereby change her initial attitude. Finally, there is the possibility that genuine changes have occurred between measurement periods. This is particularly true for properties that are highly variable, such as measures of blood pressure, temperature, and weight. The impact of these problems of stability varies depending upon the nature of the measurement and the time lapse between measurements. Obviously, some measuring instruments are more susceptible to these problems than others.

As suggested by Selltiz, et al. (1976) when there is both the possibility that the initial measure may affect the results of the second measure and the possibility of genuine changes brought about by other factors, the common practice is to try to steer a course between waiting long enough for the effects of the first testing to wear off and not long enough for a significant amount of real change to take place. There are no hard and fast rules for determining the appropriate time interval. When there is doubt, however, many investigators prefer to wait a longer rather than a shorter period of time between measurement. The outcome is then likely to be an underestimate, rather than an overestimate, of stability.

The most commonly used procedure for estimating test-retest reliability continues to be that of the Pearson product-moment correlation. As pointed out earlier, correlation procedures are not always the best methods to use and may result in inappropriate and inaccurate conclusions. A simple example should clarify this problem. Suppose that a test is administered to a random sample of five students and then readministered to the same five students after an appropriate interval. The results might be as shown in Table 8–2.

The product-moment correlation for this example is +1, which denotes perfect correlation. (Chapter 13 discusses the actual computation of this and other correlation statistics.) An investigator using this approach would then conclude that the measuring instrument, the test,

Table 8-2. Respondents' Scores on Two Tests

Test 1 at Time 1		*Test 1 at Time 2*	
Student	*Score*	*Student*	*Score*
A	100	A	50
B	90	B	40
C	80	C	30
D	70	D	20
E	70	E	20

was completely reliable. And yet, there is a great difference between the students' performance on the two tests. What has not changed from test to test, however, is the ordering of the students. Student A has the highest score on both tests, followed by students B, C, and so on, with student E earning the lowest score on both occasions. What the correlation procedure is identifying in this case is the ordering of the students. The magnitude of the scores on individual pairs between tests is ignored. If one is interested only in the consistency of ordering, then the correlation procedure is appropriate. However, if one is interested in agreement between the two sets of scores, the most appropriate approach is through the use of the Kappa statistic, which considers the magnitude of agreement (Horn and Williamson, 1977). The Kappa statistic for the above example is calculated to be 0, indicating no agreement between the scores over the two testing periods (see Fleis, 1973, for procedures). The distinction between agreement and ordering is an important one, because so much of the reliability testing reported in the literature fails to make this distinction. As can be seen from the preceding example, the investigators, as well as the readers, could be misled by an erroneous estimate of reliability.

Equivalence refers to the extent to which different instruments applied to the same individuals at the same time, or different investigators using one instrument to measure the same individuals at the same time, yield consistent results (Selltiz, et al., 1976). Under the first condition, the method of reliability most commonly discussed is *parallel* or alternate forms. The parallel forms technique appears to have been developed because of the problems inherent in the test-retest approach, that is, the problems of the time interval and learning that occur from taking the same test twice. This technique is commonly employed when repeated measures over time are desired, such as intelligence and ability tests. In the parallel method, two forms of the instrument are developed and applied to the same individuals at essentially the same time. It is assumed that each item of one form has a parallel item in the second form. Although the two forms contain different items, all items are intended to measure the same characteristics. Estimates of reliability are then determined by comparing the person's position on one measure with his position on the second (parallel) measure, using correlational statistics.

As previously noted, measures of equivalence may also be determined when comparing the results of different investigators using one instrument to measure the same individuals. This is commonly referred to as *interrater* reliability. An investigator is concerned with interrater reliability when the nature of the measurement is such that observer influence may contribute to errors of measurement. These errors may be the result of transient personal factors associated with the observer, variations in the way the instrument is administered, lack of clarity of the instrument itself, or differences in observer knowledge.

The need for interrater reliability testing is frequently encountered in nursing research. It may consist of comparing the observations of two nurses as they attempt to classify patients according to their nursing care requirements. Comparing the ratings of several observers or judges as to the quality of care provided, or the importance of selected variables on the outcome of care, would also involve interrater reliability testing.

Some elaboration of the methods for estimating the degree of reliability under these circumstances is warranted because confusion and misuse are again frequently encountered. The chi-square test, Spearman's rank correlation, and the Pearson product-moment correlation are sometimes used to analyze data for rater agreement. As will be evident after reading Chapters 12 and 13, these are measures of association and not measures of agreement. Fleiss (1973) provides a detailed illustration of the specific problems associated with using the chi-square statistic for rater agreement. The correlation coefficient measures only the extent to which two independent raters put their measurements of the same objects in the same order. As suggested by Horn and Williamson (1977), raters can be very far apart for individual measurements; but as long as they tend to rank the objects in the same order, the product-moment correlation will be high. The statistic Kappa is again recommended for use for reliability assessments between raters or observers. When Kappa is used, simple agreement between observers is corrected for chance agreement and then compared with the observer variability to assess the final significance of the observed agreement.

Another form of equivalence is sometimes referred to as *split-half* reliability. The notion here is that the measuring instrument, if long enough, can, after administration, be split into equivalent halves for the purpose of analysis. The two portions are then correlated to provide an estimate of the equivalence coefficient. Different approaches to the splitting have been taken. Some investigators suggest that odd-numbered items be compared with even-numbered items. Others suggest comparing the first half of the test with the second half. Both of these approaches, however, have severe limitations because different reliability estimates can be calculated depending upon the split. As suggested by Bohrnstedt (1970), for a 10-item scale there are 126 possible splits, all different. Some will yield reliability estimates above the true reliability, and others, below. Thus, split halves may be far from equivalent halves. Moreover, the coefficients of equivalence represent the reliability of only one-half of the original measuring instrument.

A third approach to the splitting of items considers the notion of randomness. Since all the items are intended to measure the same characteristics, a random assignment of the items to each half should be done to provide the equivalent halves. The two most common methods used for estimating split-half reliability involve Cronbach's alpha and the Kuder-Richardson formulas 20 (K-R 20) and 21 (K-R 21). For a detailed discussion of the rationale and methods, the interested reader should consult Bohrnstedt (1970) and Cronbach (1970). These methods give the average split-half correlation for all possible ways of dividing the measure into two parts and, unlike the other procedures, yield coefficients of equivalence for the full test.

The debate over the methods appropriate for split-half reliability have led to the third aspect of reliability known as homogeneity. *Homogeneity* refers to the extent to which individuals' responses to the various items or components of a measuring instrument are consistent. Rather than thinking of a measure as being divided into two halves, the notion is one of considering the homogeneity or consistency among all of the individual items of the measure. This is frequently referred to as *internal consistency*. The methods most commonly used to assess the internal consistency of a measure include the coefficient alpha and the K-R 20 and K-R 21 methods mentioned above.

Estimating the internal consistency aspect of reliability is particularly important for instruments designed to measure a particular attribute or domain of content. Many measures of job satisfaction and quality of care are examples of this type. Recalling the previous discussion of variations in scores on measuring instruments, the selection of items in an instrument may be responsible for random errors. Estimating the internal consistency of these instruments provides us with information as to the extent to which the measures are influenced by random errors due to the sampling of content. For example, if coefficient alpha proves to be very low, either the instrument is too short or the items have very little in common.

In summary, evaluating the reliability of any measurement procedure involves an estimation of the variance in scores that is attributable to unsystematic or random errors. The less the scores are influenced by these errors, the more reliable the instrument is. The more reliable the instrument is, the more consistent and dependable the results will be. Thus, the major use of the reliability coefficient is in communicating the extent to which the results obtained are repeatable. Reliability represents a basic attribute every instrument must have. Whether an investigator is using a measurement procedure developed by someone else or developing a new one, evidence of reliability must be obtained. If the instrument cannot be relied upon to yield consistent results, then the findings obtained through its application can serve no useful purpose.

It should be stressed that not all types of reliability estimates are appropriate for all measuring instruments. For example, estimating the reliability of an instrument designed to measure nitrate levels in the blood is very different from estimating the reliability of an instrument designed to measure specific attitudes. The investigator needs to know what the major sources of error are for each measurement procedure so that the most appropriate procedure for estimating reliability is selected.

VALIDITY

The validity of an instrument refers to the degree to which the instrument measures what it is intended to measure. A valid measure of the quality of nursing care should, for example, provide evidence of the qualitative nature of nursing care and not some other aspect such as housekeeping efficiency or medical treatment. Thus, the data that a measuring instrument provides should be relevant to the characteristic in which one is interested. As previously noted, estimates of validity are concerned with both constant and random errors, and validity is increased by reducing as much as possible the influence of these errors. The validity of a measuring instrument can be defined as the extent to which the differences in the scores reflect true differences among individuals on the characteristics that the researcher seeks to measure.

The subject of validity is both complex and controversial. As suggested by Kerlinger (1973), it is not possible to study validity without sooner or later inquiring into the nature and meaning of the variables. Establishing the validity of measuring instruments for certain physical properties may not be too difficult because there is little doubt about what is being measured. Establishing the validity of measuring instruments for more abstract concepts, such as the quality of nursing care, can be very difficult. Questions such as "What is nursing?" and "What is quality care?" become important and must be dealt with in some logical and orderly manner.

Although there are a variety of labels used to define the various aspects of validity, the classification of validity into three major types, as supported by The American Psychological Association (1974), appears to be the most useful and comprehensive. The three types of validity are referred to as *content, criterion-related,* and *construct.* Before discussing each of the three types, it should be recognized that all types of validity are interrelated both operationally and logically. Although many measurements require that information be obtained on all three types, the central purpose to which the investigator intends to apply the instrument should dictate the specific type of evidence of validity to be investigated. If, for example, the investigator is interested in developing a measure of nursing performance to predict nurses' ability to function effectively in the emergency room, then evidence of predictive validity, a form of criterion-related validity, would be important.

Content validity refers to the ability of the instrument adequately to represent the domain of content being considered. For example, an investigator interested in measuring the level of job satisfaction among nurses' or clients' satisfaction with nursing care would want initially to be assured that the items of the instrument are representative of the universe of items relevant to job satisfaction or client satisfaction. In principle, this requires that the universe of the behavior in question be completely specified and all the items appropriate to its measurement be enumerated. In practice, however, this is often impossible. In some cases the number of items may approach infinity, and in others the number of items may be unknown. What the investigator can do is to define precisely the behavior in question and, through a search of the literature, determine how the concept has been used. For example, the concept of job satisfaction may be identified not as a single concept but rather as a multidimensional concept including such aspects as pay, promotion, coworkers, and supervision. Thus, a series of items can be constructed to measure each of these substrata within the domain of job satisfaction. As noted by Bohrnstedt (1970), the measuring instruments show content validity to the degree that items sampled from the domain of content are representative of all strata and that items tap the subtleties of meaning within each of the strata.

Content validity has no empirical basis; that is, no single content validity coefficient can be computed. Logical and statistical procedures, however, can be applied to help ensure that items have content validity. Although content validity does rely on judgment, the notion of content validity should not be equated with face validity. Face validity refers to nothing more than the subjective judgment that the measure or instrument looks like it is related to the concept of interest. While face validity may be useful as a point of departure in the development or assessment of an instrument, it provides an insufficient basis for inference and should never be used alone as a measure of validity.

Several steps can be taken to help ensure the representation of the various aspects and meanings of the concept that one is interested in measuring. It is the evidence that the researcher has proceeded through these steps that supports the conclusion that a measure or instrument has content validity. First, the domain can be stratified into its major components. A careful review of the literature will assist in identifying the most important and obvious meanings or facets of the concept necessary for the stratification. Second, several items can be constructed to represent the shades of meaning associated with each stratum. Third, after data have been collected, correlations can be computed to determine if the items within a stratum correlate more highly with each other than they do with items in other strata. Bohrnstedt (1970) provides a description of the use of this analysis for content validity, as does Nunnally (1978).

Criterion-related validity refers to the extent to which the instrument corresponds to some other observation, the criterion, that measures accurately the phenomena of interest. Both *concurrent* and *predictive* validity are recognized as subcategories of criterion-related validity. Concurrent validity is established by comparing the measure of interest with some other measure designed for the same purpose. Predictive validity is established by determining how well the measure predicts some future behavior. The distinction between these two aspects is important. Concurrent validity reflects only the status quo at a particular time. For example, an investigator may wish to distinguish between persons who have high blood pressure and those who do not. A test that helps distinguish those individuals who differ in their present status is said to have concurrent validity. Predictive validity, on the other hand, involves a time interval during which something may happen; that is, nurses are trained, students take an exam, or patients develop a disease. Thus, another investigator may wish to predict which people are likely to become hypertensive. The adequacy of the test for distinguishing people who will differ in the future is called its predictive validity.

Criterion-related validity is demonstrated by a single coefficient, and both correlational procedures and measures of agreement are used to estimate the extent of validity. The cautions associated with correlation statistics, discussed earlier under reliability, are equally applicable for validity testing. The reader is reminded of the differences between measures of association and measures of agreement.

Obtaining an appropriate criterion measure is not always easy. If there were some other measure that provided us with a person's true position on the variable of interest, there would often be no need for another measure of the variable, unless the available method of measurement was either too expensive or for some reason impractical or inappropriate to use. In the absence of a valid criterion, investigators must select what seems to be the most appropriate criterion. Determining a near-zero correlation between the new measure and the criterion measure, then, does not necessarily justify immediate dismissal of the new measure as invalid. Further testing with other criteria, along with the pursuit of evidence toward content and construct validity, would be appropriate. As sometimes happens, the new measure may in turn become the criterion for future testing situations.

Construct validity involves the assembling of empirical evidence to support the inference that a particular measure has meaning. Construct validity becomes important and appropriate when there is no criterion or universe of content that can be accepted as adequate to define the phenomena to be measured. Examination of construct validity involves validation not only of the measuring instrument but of the theory underlying it. In other words, the measuring instrument is related to an overall theoretical framework in order to determine whether the instrument is tied to the concepts and theoretical assumptions that are employed.

The theoretical notions one has about the property being measured lead the investigator to postulate various kinds and degrees of relationships between the property and other specified variables. In order to demonstrate construct validity, an investigator has to show that these relationships do in fact hold.

The most common approach to construct validity is known as the multitrait-multimethod approach developed by Campbell and Fiske (1970). This involves two types of validation: *convergent* validation and *discriminant* validation. Convergent validation involves confirmation of a relationship by independent measurement procedures. In other words, different methods of measuring the same procedure should yield similar results. Operationally, this means that the correlation coefficients among scores for a given property measured by two or more instruments should be high. The higher the separate measures correlate with each other, the greater the convergent validity. Discriminant validity refers to evidence that the construct as measured can be differentiated from other constructs. In other words, correlating two measures that represent different constructs should yield lower correlations than those between measures of the same construct.

The multitrait-multimethod approach involves the development of a correlation matrix, a procedure explained in detail by Campbell and Fiske (1970). Factor analysis may also be used to provide evidence of construct validity, by identifying the internal consistency of a set of variables proposed to measure a construct. The place of factor analysis in the establishment of validity is well documented by Nunnally (1978).

It should be apparent that construct validity cannot adequately be tested by any single procedure; it requires evidence from a number of sources and is a matter of degree rather than an all-or-none property. Construct validation, and, in fact, all types of validation, should be viewed as a continuing process. It is generally agreed that most measures dealing with anything less than concrete phenomena should be kept under surveillance to see if, through time, they continue to behave as they should (Nunnally, 1978).

RELATIONSHIP BETWEEN RELIABILITY AND VALIDITY

Understanding the relationship between reliability and validity is important for a clear recognition of both the meanings implied and the differences between the two concepts.

Reliability relates to the concepts of consistency or repeatability. The reliability of an instrument or measurement procedure refers to the degree to which the instrument can be depended upon to yield consistent results upon repeated applications. *Validity* refers to the ability of the instrument to measure what it seeks to measure.

Reliability is a necessary condition for validity. Stated another way, one cannot have validity unless one has reliability. An instrument that cannot be depended upon to give the same results upon repetition obviously cannot be used to measure accurately and therefore cannot have any validity (Suchman, 1967). This fact does not imply, however, that a reliable measure is valid. One can have a highly reliable instrument, but it may not be measuring what one wants it to measure. For example, the method used to measure serum cholesterol level in the blood may be shown to be highly reliable; that is, upon repeated applications on the same person over a short period of time, the serum cholesterol level remains unchanged. But to suggest that serum cholesterol level is a valid measure of coronary artery disease is, of course, erroneous.

While perhaps far removed from the health care field, one further illustration should serve to exemplify the differences between the concepts of reliability and validity. Suppose there are three rifles, each solidly fixed and aimed at the bull's-eye of a target. Figures 8–2, 8–3, and 8–4 illustrate the targets after equal numbers of rounds have been fired from each rifle.

In Figure 8–2, while one shot hit the bull's-eye, the rest are scattered all over the target board. Figure 8–3 shows the shots to be closely spaced together but not on or near the bull's-eye, while in Figure 8–4,

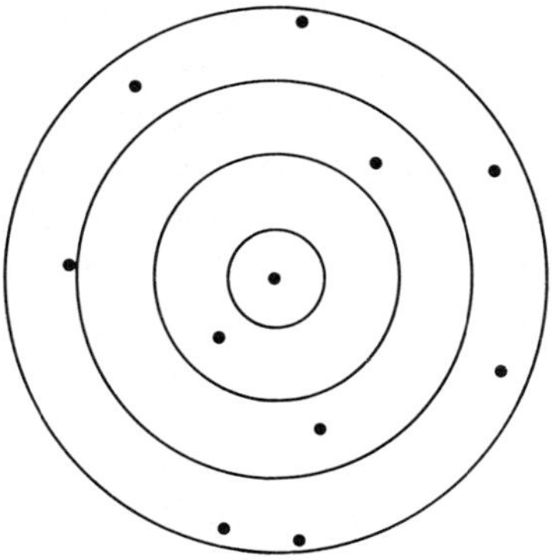

Figure 8-2. Shots fired from first rifle.

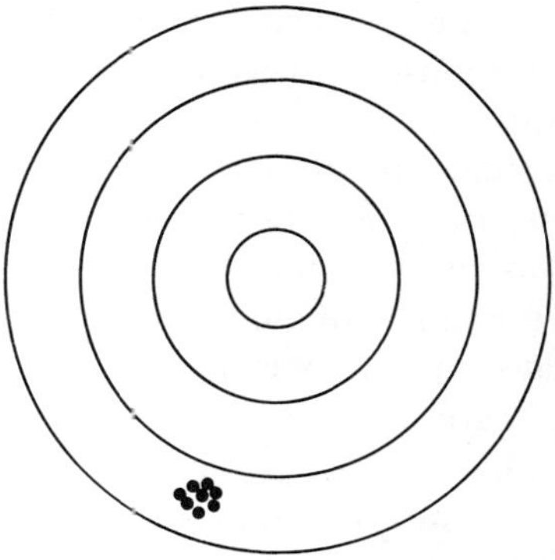

Figure 8-3. Shots fired from second rifle.

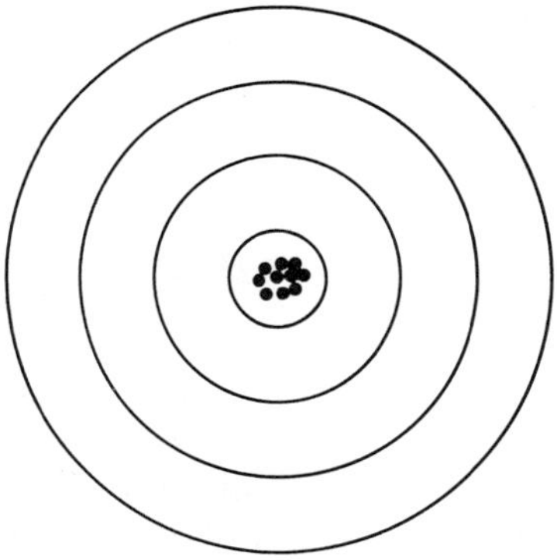

Figure 8-4. Shots fired from third rifle.

the shots are both close together and within the intended bull's-eye. Obviously, in Figure 8–2 a great deal of variability is observed; the weapon used could hardly be called upon to yield consistent results. The weapon used in Figure 8–3 shows little variability, as the shots are all close together. While this rifle illustrates the properties of high reliability, the shots are far from the intended target. Figure 8–3 thus illustrates high reliability without validity. Finally, Figure 8–4 clearly illustrates high reliability and validity. The third weapon yields consistent results, and it is doing what it is intended to do, that is, shooting bullets into the area of the bull's-eye.

In addition to the characteristics of reliability and validity, the measurement process also needs to be evaluated in terms of its *sensitivity* and *appropriateness*. *Sensitivity* refers to the ability of the instrument to make distinctions fine enough for the purposes that it is to serve. For example, a crude measure of patient satisfaction that distinguishes only two positions, satisfied and unsatisfied, is unlikely to reveal important shifts in satisfaction resulting from some change in the provision of care. The investigator should consider whether the lack of differences found after the administration of a measuring instrument indicates that there really was no change, or that there was change but the instrument was too insensitive to detect it. Adding more categories to the measurement does not necessarily solve the problem of insensitivity. The added categories must genuinely tap the added distinctions.

Appropriateness refers to the extent to which the measuring instrument is relevant for the respondents. Patient satisfaction questionnaires again serve as an example. The question of concern to an investigator is whether or not clients or patients really have the knowledge necessary to offer an opinion or attitude concerning the variable of interest. Although there is no simple solution to this problem, the investigator should be alert to its existence. Asking questions or including items that reveal the clients' knowledge may enlighten the investigator as to whether or not the respondents are familiar with the topic and can thus be expected to have opinions about it.

SUMMARY

In summary, this chapter has discussed a number of aspects central to the measurement of variables. Measurement itself was defined as the assignment of numbers to objects or events, or properties of objects or events, according to a set of rules. Rules were identified as the most significant component of the measurement procedure because they can determine the quality of measurement. Four scales, or levels, of measurement were discussed: nominal, ordinal, interval, and ratio. It was pointed out that the operations that may be performed on a given set of numbers, and thus the inferences that can be made about the data, are dependent upon the level of measurement, or the type of scale, developed.

A number of factors affecting both the characteristics being measured and the process of measurement were identified and discussed. The impact of these factors in terms of random or constant error led to the discussion of reliability and validity of the measuring instrument. Finally, the reader was introduced to the notion that all measuring instruments need to be evaluated in terms of their reliability, validity, sensitivity, and appropriateness.

BIBLIOGRAPHY

American Psychological Association. *Standards for Educational and Psychological Tests.* Washington: American Psychological Association, 1974.

Bohrnstedt, G.W. Reliability and validity assessment in attitude measurement, in Summers, G. (Ed.), *Attitude Measurement.* Chicago: Rand McNally and Company, 1970, p. 80.

Campbell, D. T., & Fiske, W. Convergent and discrimanent validation by the multitrait-multimethod matrix, in Summers, G. (Ed.), *Attitude Measurement.* Chicago: Rand McNally and Company, 1970, Chapter 4.

Cronbach, L. J. *Essentials of Psychological Testing,* 3rd edition. New York: Harper & Row, 1970.

Fleiss, L. J. *Statistical Methods for Rates and Proportions.* New York: John Wiley & Sons, 1973, p. 140.

Horn, S. D. & Williamson, J. W. Statistical methods for reliability and validity testing: An application to nominal group judgments in health care. *Medical Care* 1977, *15,* No. 11.

Kerlinger, F. N. *Foundations of Behavioral Research,* 2nd edition. New York: Holt, Rinehart & Winston, Inc., 1973.

Nunnally, J. C. *Psychometric Theory.* 2nd edition. New York: McGraw-Hill Book Co., 1978.

Selltiz, G., Wrightsman, L. S., & Cook, S. W. *Research Methods in Social Relations,* 3rd edition. New York: Holt, Rinehart & Winston, 1976, p. 181.

Suchman, E. A. *Evaluative Research, Principles and Practice in Public Service and Social Action Programs.* New York: Russell Sage Foundation, 1967, p. 116.

9
Sampling Techniques

Phyllis Giovannetti

Most of the knowledge, attitudes, and opinions that we accumulate throughout life are based on samples. We frequently come to conclusions about people in general or about particular ethnic groups based on association with perhaps a very small number of people. Sometimes these opinions come not from personal experience but from what is heard from others. A one-time experience with a warm and caring nurse during a childhood illness has motivated more than one young woman to select a career in nursing. Eating one bad olive or, for that matter, twenty good ones at one sitting has precipitated many an "I hate olives" statement. Most people have had a good deal of experience with sampling. However, it should be apparent after assimilating this chapter that much of the knowledge, attitudes, and opinions come from very inadequate samples. The common statement that "first impressions are lasting impressions" is in direct opposition to the theory of sampling that does not generally condone samples of one. Increasing the sample size does not necessarily improve the situation. Eating an entire jar of rotten olives hardly gives the good ones a chance to impress our palate.

Although experiences with sampling may not have incorporated the principles and procedures of good sampling, they provide the student with a background understanding of sampling for research studies. Common sense is a basic prerequisite for understanding the topic. This is not to suggest that the concepts and aspects of sampling are simple. Quite the contrary, for there are many aspects of sampling that are both complex and technical. The purpose of this chapter, then, is to present material related to the purposes, definitions, and concepts of sampling. Types of samples and procedures for sampling along with sample size and nonsampling errors, are shown through use of hypothetical examples. Although a number of textbooks have been written entirely on the subject of sampling, by the end of this chapter the student will have gained sufficient knowledge, skills, and confidence to draw samples for a research study.

PURPOSE OF A SAMPLE

Sampling consists of obtaining information from a portion of a larger group. The major purpose of sampling is to make some estimation or inference about the total group from which the sample has been selected. The practice of sampling is common, and there are many reasons for obtaining samples rather than observing the larger group.

The use of samples is almost always less expensive and more expedient than using the entire population or complete census counts. For example, if the American Nurses Association were interested in interviewing its members regarding some policy decision, it would take many months to locate each of its members and complete the interviews. The costs of interviewing, travel, and data processing time would be exhorbitant. Instead, a well-designed sample of 5% of the membership could provide essentially the same information and require only a small portion of the cost of interviewing the entire membership. Such a project would be feasible, whereas a study of the population would be prohibitive.

In addition, samples may be more accurate than complete census counts. A very large survey employing interviewing, for example, would require an enormous staff of interviewers. The result might be that the overall quality of the interviews would be difficult to control and could be lower than that obtained by a small, well-trained group of interviewers. In addition, a smaller scale study would permit more attention to follow-up procedures, thereby increasing the number of completed interviews. The length of time in the interviewing period may also affect the accuracy of the data. If the period were lengthy, it would be difficult, if not impossible, to specify to what point in time the data refer. While this problem is inherent in any interviewing project that is executed over time, the seriousness of the problem grows with the duration of the interviewing period (Babbie, 1973).

In some instances samples must be used; there are no alternatives. The taking of blood samples provides an excellent example. Few would argue with a technician that a very small sample of blood is sufficient to give a precise picture of the nature and content of the red and white blood cells. We are fortunate indeed that a sample is all that is required.

Teachers give examinations to sample the knowledge of students. There is no other way of measuring all that a student has learned. A chocolate factory would go out of business if every cordial had to be squeezed to determine the consistency of the center.

BASIC DEFINITIONS AND CONCEPTS

Before discussing the various types of sampling techniques and procedures, some basic definitions and concepts should be explained. As previously noted, samples are used to represent some larger group. The larger group is referred to as the *target population;* it includes all the cases which meet a designated set of criteria. For example, a target population may be all nurses in the United States, with nurses referring to RNs only and United States referring to citizens only. Similarly, all graduates of a particular university or all patients admitted to a hospital during a specified period of time may be defined as the target population of a sampling study. The target population need not be people. It may consist of all the nursing tasks performed for a specified group of patients, all of the operating rooms in university teaching hospitals of 500 beds or more, all of the records on file at a community health center, or all of the incoming telephone calls occurring within a specified period of time.

One population may be included in another population. For example, the population of all the cases of hepatitis reported in a particular city is included in the population of all cases of hepatitis reported in the state. In this instance, the included population is referred to as a *subpopulation,* or a *population stratum.* A population may be subdivided into a number of strata, each of which represents mutually exclusive segments of the population. A researcher may be interested in a target population which has been divided into one or more strata, or may wish to treat a specified stratum as the target population itself without reference to its inclusion in a larger population.

A *sampling element,* or *population element,* refers to a single member of the population. For example, in the population of RNs in the United States, the sampling elements are individual RNs in the United States. It is important to define the population clearly so that the sampling elements can be identified. The definition of the sampling elements must always state which elements are included in or excluded from the target population (Williams, 1978). In a study of United States RNs, the definition of an RN would need to be specified. Would it mean RNs who also happen to have a master's or doctoral degree? Would it include RNs from three-year programs, two-year programs, employed fulltime or parttime, or not employed? Similarly, the term "United States" must be defined. Does it refer to citizens, or residents, or both? What about those who are out of the country during the study period? Obviously, the target population of United States RNs requires a very precise definition before a sample can be drawn.

A *sampling unit* refers to the element or set of elements considered for selection in some stage of the sampling procedure. In a simple, one-stage sample, the sampling units are the same as the sampling elements. In more complex samples, different sampling units can be identified. For example, a researcher may select a sample of hospitals within an area, then select a sample of wards within the selected hospitals, and finally select a sample of patients from the selected wards. The sampling units for these three stages of sampling are hospitals, wards, and patients, of which only the last of these, the patients, are the elements.

A *sampling frame* refers to the actual list of sampling units from which the sample is selected. If a sample of patients is selected from a hospital's inpatient register, the register is the sampling frame. In this case, the population is also the register of hospital inpatients. The relationship between populations and sampling frame is important. Samples drawn from a sampling frame provide information appropriate for describing the population of elements that comprise the sampling frame. A sample of nurses selected from a list of nurses who are members of the State Nurses' Association can be used to describe a population defined as nurses who belong to the State Nurses' Association. The sample cannot be used to describe all nurses within the state, for we know that not all nurses belong to the State Association.

Not all research investigations can make use of a prepared list of population elements. In many instances, the researchers must prepare a sampling frame, and the formulation of such a frame requires very clear and precise definitions of the population units.

Sampling error refers to sampling variability or the difference between sample estimates of a population value and the true population value. Regardless of the type of sampling procedure selected, sampling errors occur. The vagaries of chance create the situation. Even when two samples are drawn randomly from exactly the same population in exactly the same manner, the two samples will almost always differ. Later in this chapter it will become evident that with probability sampling procedures the investigator can calculate the degree of sampling error to be expected for a given sample design. When using nonprobability sampling procedures, however, the investigator has no mathematically defined way of estimating the potential sampling error.

SAMPLING TYPES AND PROCEDURES

Once a target population from which a sample will be drawn has been determined, the problem is to decide how to select the sample. The importance of the selection method cannot be underestimated as it has a direct bearing on the inferences that can be made about the population. Let us assume that a research instructor wanted to sample 10 students from the class. The most expedient way might be to choose the first 10 students sitting in the front row of the class. However, if the instructor were interested in the average height of the students, for example, it is doubtful that this sample would adequately reflect the properties of the target population. It may be that all of the short students sit up front to avoid craning their necks to see the board. A sample of students taken from the front row could thus be biased in favor of the short students. If the instructor, in anticipation of this possibility, avoided the error by eliminating the front row of students altogether the problem would not be solved, because the bias would then tend to be in the opposite direction. Furthermore, the instructor might be mistaken in her hypothesis, and there might be no short students at all in the front row.

The sampling biases that may invade the sampling procedure are not usually known at the time the sample is being collected. Moreover, information about a number of variables is frequently obtained at one time. While there is no doubt that for some purposes the crude method of sampling the front row of students would be perfectly adequate, we have no way of ensuring that it is adequate for all the variables of interest unless our sampling method is such that no possibility of a bias can arise.

The many sampling procedures that are employed can be classified according to two general types: *probability sampling procedures* and *nonprobability sampling procedures*. Probability sampling procedures are those aimed at eliminating the opportunity for bias to occur. Nonprobability sampling procedures can offer no such guarantee.

Probability Sampling

Probability sampling is distinguished from nonprobability sampling by random selection. Random selection means that the sample is obtained in such a manner that every possible sample has a specific probability of being selected. Thus, one can specify for every element in the target population the probability that it will be included in the sample.

There are a number of very important advantages that accrue with the use of probability sampling procedures. First, because the investigator can determine the probability of selection for each element of the population, a sample that is more representative of the target population than that obtained by other sampling procedures is more likely to occur. Both conscious and unconscious selection biases are avoided. Second, probability samples provide the investigator with the information necessary to estimate the magnitude of the sampling error. Recall that sampling error refers to the difference between a population value (such as the average weight of a target population of newborns) and a sample value (such as the average weight of a sample of newborns taken from the target population). It is unlikely that a sample will contain no sampling error, but probability sampling does permit an estimate of the degree of expected error. Third, with probability samples, inferential statistical techniques can be used with greater confidence.

The stated advantages of probability sampling might suggest that samples not collected in this manner have no place in the research field. Although probability sampling should be a goal of all investigators, the achievement of such a goal is not always possible. In many instances, probability samples are expensive and inconvenient, and some studies simply could not be done if adherence to probability sampling were demanded.

Finally, it should be noted that biases may enter into the selection of sampling elements even when probability sampling procedures are used. For example, an investigator may select randomly a sample to respond to a questionnaire, but for one reason or another, some people may refuse to participate. If certain segments of the population systematically refuse to participate, the sample could be biased by nonresponse errors.

Several probability sampling procedures are common: *simple random sampling, systematic sampling, stratified sampling,* and *cluster sampling.*

Simple random sampling refers to the process of sampling that gives each element in the population an equal and nonzero chance of being included in the sample. Moreover, it makes the selection of every possible combination of the desired number of cases equally likely. The usual procedure for the selection of a random sample involves the use of a list of random numbers. Such lists are frequently found in textbooks of statistics and represent sets of numbers that have been shown to have no evidence of systematic order.

To make use of a table of random numbers, it is first necessary to number all the elements in the population under study. The investigator then, in a random fashion, selects a number from the table. This frequently is accomplished by a blind pencil stab at the page. That number becomes the first case in the sample. One can then proceed down the column of numbers on the random table until the desired sample size is collected. The investigator choses each case from the population or sampling frame that has the number corresponding to the number selected from the table. An important theoretical issue is whether a sample element is to be eligible for selection into a sample only once or is to be replaced in the pool for possible reselection into the sample. The first option is referred to as sampling without replacement and the second, sampling with replacement. With finite populations the usual practice is to sample without replacement, that is, with each sample element having the opportunity of being selected only once. Thus, if a duplicate number is selected from a table of random numbers, it is ignored (Warwick, 1975).

Systematic sampling refers to the procedure of selecting every k^{th} element of the population after the first element is selected randomly from the first k sampling elements. The procedure for selecting a systematic sample is operationally very simple. Suppose an investigator is interested in obtaining some information from adult members of a local Health Maintenance Organization (HMO), and a list of 1000 such members is available. For a sample of 100, the interval k would be 10($k = N/n = 1000/100 = 10$). That is, to obtain a sample of 100 from a population of 1000, every tenth individual must be selected. In keeping with our definition, however, selection of the first element must be done using a random procedure; and it must be selected from the first k sampling elements, which in the present example is 10. From a list of random numbers between 1 and 10, suppose the number 8 was selected. The sample then would consist of individuals numbered 8, 18, 28, 38, and so on to the one hundredth case numbered 998.

Systematic sampling is included as a probability sampling procedure as long as a random starting point is used to select the first sampling element. Thus, it is ensured that each element in the population has an equal probability of being included in the sample. Additional considerations, however, are also important. When selecting systematic sampling as the procedure of choice, it is essential that the order of the listing of population elements be random with respect to the measurement of interest. This is necessary to avoid the possibility that the selection interval and the data have the same cycle. For example, if the list of HMO members were made up of husbands and wives who appear alternately on successive lines, then a systematic sample with an even-numbered selection interval would consist of either all males or all females.

A systematic sample of households also serves well to illustrate this point. Suppose that every tenth house in a subdivision has been selected for a survey to determine the average income of a community. If the first house selected is a corner house, every tenth house may also be a corner house. It is quite possible that the incomes of families who own corner lots are quite different from those who do not. It could, of course, be that no corner houses are selected. Although the average income would be very different, the effect would be the same: a grossly biased sample of average income. It is important, therefore, to be aware of how the listing of the population elements is derived because systematic patterns of behaviors are not always obvious.

It should be evident that systematic sampling and simple random sampling are virtually identical, and the choice of one method in favor of the other generally is based on consideration of convenience. Drawing a simple random sample of 100 from a list of random numbers can be a laborious process, whereas a systematic sample of 100 could be obtained very quickly.

Stratified sampling refers to the procedure of dividing the population of interest into one or more mutually exclusive subgroups (called strata) and then randomly selecting elements from each group. Whereas simple random sampling and systematic sampling represent two alternatives for selecting a sample from a list, stratified sampling represents a modification of the sampling frame. Many research studies lend themselves to stratified sampling, and use of the procedure often can be an improvement over simple random or systematic sampling.

Consider a target population of nine nurses: three associate degree graduates, three diploma graduates, and three baccalaureate graduates. Let us assume that we are interested in selecting a sample of three. Using simple random sampling, it is obvious that the sample may not represent one or even two of the different educational programs. The sample could consist of all three diploma graduates, or perhaps two diploma graduates and one baccalaureate graduate. It is quite possible, in fact highly probable, that any sample selected using simple random selection would not be representative of the three educational levels. Looking again at our target population, three different homogeneous groups or subsets can be identified: associate degree graduates, diploma graduates, and baccalaureate graduates. There is no variation among the members within each group with respect to educational preparation. Using stratified sampling, one nurse from each of the three groups is selected. (In actual practice it is likely our population size would be larger.) The function of stratification, then, is to organize the target population into homogeneous groups. The population elements within each group are as similar to each other as possible (homogeneity within groups), and among groups they are as different from each other as possible (heterogeneity between groups). In this way appropriate representation of the diverse elements within the population is assured.

The selection of variables for stratification depends upon the availability of variables and the purpose of the investigation. Very often, variables such as age and sex are used to stratify a population because they frequently are available and related to other variables. The researcher should, however, be concerned primarily with those variables that presumably are related to the variables of interest. For example, a researcher interested in the care provided to nursing home patients might well stratify the nursing homes according to size, type of ownership, and levels of care offered.

It is not necessary to sample the same number of elements from each stratum. In many cases, stratifying the population will divide the population into unequal subgroups. From a population of nursing personnel employed full time at a number of health agencies, let us assume that 70 percent are RNs, 20 percent LPNs, and 10 percent aides. In this instance the researcher may decide to select subjects in proportion to the size of the stratum. Thus, a proportional stratified sample of 100 nursing personnel would consist of 70 RNs, 20 LPNs, and 10 aides.

Cluster sampling refers to the sampling technique in which the elements for the sample are chosen from the population in groups or clusters rather than singly. Frequently, in large-scale studies, an investigator is unable to obtain a reliable list of all the elements within a target population, and therefore construction of such a list would be prohibitively expensive. In such instances the three preceding procedures for sampling from lists of elements are not appropriate. Cluster sampling provides a technique for the selection of samples from populations that cannot easily be listed.

Consider an investigator interested in certain traits of patients hospitalized for myocardial infarction (MI). A complete list of all patients currently hospitalized for the condition would undoubtedly be difficult, if not impossible, to obtain. It is often the case, however, that lists of subpopulations containing the population elements do exist or can be created practically. In the above example, patients with myocardial infarction can be identified within hospitals, and a list of hospitals can be obtained or easily created. The hospitals would be referred to as the clusters, and the sampling elements would be those patients hospitalized for myocardial infarction. The list of hospitals would be sampled using a simple random, systematic, or stratified sampling technique. The next step would be to sample from lists of MI patients in each of the selected hospitals; again, one of the three previously discussed techniques could be used. Even if a master list of all patients currently hospitalized for myocardial infarction were available, economic and administrative considerations would be likely to dictate the use of the cluster sampling.

Just how a cluster is defined depends on the unit of enquiry. In the preceding example the hospitals were identified as the clusters, since they contained patients and the patients were the unit of enquiry. If the hospitals were the unit of enquiry, some larger aggregate such as cities or counties would be designated as the clusters. Generally, more precise results are obtained when clusters are identified as heterogeneous groups, that is, when there is no variation from cluster to cluster and all of the variability in the population is within the cluster. In the previous example, it might be assumed that "patient traits" were not unique to any one state or even any particular hospital. Thus each cluster could be assumed to be similar. Had the investigator been interested in the *treatment* of myocardial infarction, however, such an assumption would probably be challenged because hospitals could vary in their approach to such treatment. Recall that in stratified sampling, the reverse situation prevailed; strata were identified as containing homogeneous units.

A common extension of cluster sampling is known as *multistage sampling*. Rather than the sampling of entire clusters, the sample is selected in two or more steps or stages. The procedure is useful when the population units are arranged in hierarchical groups. A survey of hospitals might be conducted by random selection of states, counties within those states, and hospitals within those counties. In this three-stage sampling scheme, the states would be considered the primary sampling units, the counties the secondary units, and the hospitals the tertiary units.

Although cluster and multistage sampling techniques have important advantages in the areas of economic and administrative efficiency, they can result in larger sampling errors. A simple random sample is subject to a single sampling error, whereas a two-stage cluster sample is subject to two sampling errors. The first sample of clusters represents the population of clusters only within a range of sampling error. The sample of elements selected from within a sampled cluster represents all the elements of that cluster only within a range of sampling error. In a household survey, for example, the investigator runs a certain risk of selecting a sample of disproportionately poor city blocks plus a sample of disproportionately poor households within those blocks. This problem can be partially compensated for by increasing the sample size at each stage of the sampling process. In fact, it is usually more efficient economically to have a small sample size in the first stage of selection followed by a larger sample size in the final stage. As previously noted, sampling error can also be minimized by increasing the homogeneity of the elements being sampled, and the best method of doing this is to use a stratified sampling technique at each stage of cluster sampling.

Nonprobability Sampling

Nonprobability sampling procedures refer to those methods of sampling that do not permit one to specify the probability of selection for each element in the population. Thus, some elements in the population may have a greater or lesser chance than others of being selected into the sample. This situation can occur in all probability sampling procedures except simple random sampling, but an important distinction exists. With probability sampling procedures, the investigator can specify the exact probability of selection for each population element. With nonprobability sampling procedures, the magnitude of the different probabilities is unknown. Nonprobability samples are not necessarily inaccurate; the problem is that a measurement of the sample accuracy is not possible. There is a further important aspect of nonprobability sampling—there is no assurance that every element in the population even has a chance of being selected; that is, the probability of selection for some population elements may be zero.

The limitations of nonprobability sampling are obvious. If the probability of selection is unknown and if there is no assurance that every element within the target population has a chance of being selected, the investigator cannot be sure that the sample is representative of the target population. This is a severe restriction indeed when the purpose of the sample is to make generalizations about the population from which it came.

Despite the obvious limitations of nonprobability sampling procedures, they are used frequently in nursing research as well as in much of the research in the behavioral sciences. Their advantages stem from the fact that they are often more convenient and less costly and, in some cases, the only approach available. When generalizability of research findings is not a goal, as in the case of some exploratory studies and investigation of the relationship between variables, nonprobability samples are appropriate and in some cases even preferred.

Once having decided to use a nonprobability sample, the investigator must take special care in defining the target population, selecting the sample, and relating conclusions and inferences drawn from the study. Since nonprobability sampling involves, at some stage, subjective choice of the sampling elements, the term *judgment sampling* is sometimes used.

Three nonprobability sampling procedures are common: *accidental sampling, quota sampling,* and *purposive sampling.*

Accidental sampling, or *convenience sampling,* refers to the procedure of selecting the sample from the subjects that happen to be available. An accidental sample might include all the students in a classroon, all the patients who happen to be in the hospital on a particular day, or all mothers who were delivered by a nurse midwife during a one-month period. The procedure is often employed by the news media. The first 20 people who happen to walk by an interviewer and are willing to be interviewed become the basis for such statements as "four out of five persons are in favor of a new City Hall."

There is no way of knowing what biases might be introduced by accidental samples unless, of course, a parallel study using a probability sample or a complete census were conducted at the same time. The available subjects may be typical or atypical of the population with respect to the variables of interest. If the population is fairly homogeneous with respect to these variables, the potential risks may be minimal. With heterogeneous populations, however, the biases can be great, and the use of this sampling procedure should be carefully scrutinized. Accidental sampling represents the weakest form of nonprobability sampling, yet the procedure continues to be commonly used.

Many nursing research studies have been conducted using accidental samples. Consider a study of primary nursing care assignment. A nursing unit practicing primary nursing is selected for study and compared with another unit where the new nursing modality has not been implemented. Both nursing units may be considered accidental or convenience samples. In many instances there simply are no feasible alternatives to the selection of such a sample. With reasonable knowledge and care, and full realization of the limitations imposed upon the generalizability of the findings, the procedure can be useful in advancing the science and practice of nursing. The importance of clearly defining the characteristics of the population or the setting from which the sample was selected, and the need for study replications, should be obvious whenever accidental samples are used.

Quota sampling is similar to accidental sampling in that the population elements that are readily available are selected, but an additional step is taken to ensure the inclusion of diverse elements of the population. The goal of quota sampling is the selection of a sample that is roughly proportional to the population on a few demographic variables of concern. Knowledge of the characteristics of the population is thus important and is used as the basis for establishing the quotas. For example, if it is known that 20 percent of the population served by an ambulatory care center are male, then the nonprobability sample should be collected in such a way that 20 percent of the sample represents males. Rather than selecting the first 100 clients who arrive at the center, as for an accidental sample, the investigator would deliberately select arrivals until the sample size of 100 consisted of 20% males. In other words, the investigator would continue with the selection of clients until the quota of 80 females and 20 males was fulfilled.

Let us assume that the research question relates to attitude toward the use of nurse practitioners. Let us further assume that females prefer to be seen by nurse practitioners, while males prefer to be seen by physicians. If the investigator selected an accidental sample, it is quite possible that less than 20 percent of the sample would be males. Analysis of the predominantly female sample would lead one to believe that the population was overwhelmingly in favor of nurse practitioners. On tbe other hand, if a quota sample were used to ensure male representation, the true viewpoint of the population would be more likely to be determined.

Although the researcher may try to obtain a sample with components that are proportional to the corresponding strata of the target population, in practice, the final sample may not have the exact proportion desired. There are a number of reasons for this. If questionnaires are used, the return rate might be different for each segment of the population. If interviews are used, the interviewers may not carry out their instructions exactly, or the intended number of cases may not present themselves within the alloted time. Whatever the reason, investigators frequently end up with a quota sample that does not contain the proportions intended. The inadequacy of the sample, however, can be corrected in the analysis by weighing the different strata in terms of their proportion in the population (Chein, 1976).

Consider the hypothetical data in Table 9-1, which represent the results of a sample of 1,000 women interviewed regarding the adequacy of their prenatal preparation for labor. The table shows that 500 (50%) of these women interviewed were cared for by nurse midwives and 500 (50%) were cared for by physicians. Suppose it is known that for this particular target population from a community served by a large teaching hospital, 25% of the women are serviced by nurse midwives while the remaining 75% are serviced by physicians. If the intention were only to report the figures for each group of women separately, there would be no need to make an adjustment. For example, it could be reported that of 500 women cared for by nurse midwives, 400, or 80%, felt that they had been adequately prepared for labor. On the other hand, if we wanted to estimate the proportion of the target

Table 9-1. Hypothetical Responses of Clients Serviced by Nurse Midwives and Physicians Regarding the Adequacy of Their Preparation for Labor[a]

	Serviced by		
Adequacy of Preparation	*Nurse Midwife*	*Physician*	*Total*
Adequately prepared	400	200	600
Inadequately prepared	100	300	400
	500	500	1000

[a] Sample: $n = 1{,}000$.

population that felt their preparation was adequate, the sample findings would be misleading. Table 9-1 reveals that 600, or 60%, felt that their preparation was adequate. But the sample overrepresented the nurse midwife group and underrepresented the physician group. An estimate of the correct figure for the total population must consider what the responses would have been if only 25% of the sample contained the nurse midwife clients. A simple way of doing this is to multiply the responses of the nurse midwife group by 0.5 (to reduce the 50% to 25%) and the physician group by 1.5 (to increase the 50% to 75%). Table 9-2 provides the weighted response rates.

It is now evident that only 50% of the target population, as compared with the unweighted estimate of 60%, consider their preparation for labor adequate. By weighting the strata according to their actual proportions in the population, we have attempted to provide a better estimate of the population.

From the preceding example, it is evident that if the sample does not

Table 9-2. Hypothetical Weighted Response Rates of Clients Serviced by Nurse Midwives and Physicians Regarding Adequacy of Preparation for Labor[a]

	Serviced by		
Adequacy of Preparation	*Nurse Midwife*	*Physicians*	*Total*
Adequately prepared	200	300	500
Inadequately prepared	50	450	500
	250	750	1000

[a]Sample: $n = 1{,}000$.

contain the exact quotas as planned, the sample can be adjusted at the time of analysis. The adjustments, however, can be made only if the sample contains enough cases from each stratum to make possible an estimate of the population stratum value. If the sample were collected without consideration of diverse elements within the target population, it is quite possible that the sample would contain too few cases of the diverse elements to permit an estimate of the population.

Quota sampling implies that the diverse elements or characteristics of the population that are of major importance to the study question are known. Frequently, such characteristics as age, sex, education, socioeconomic status, and ethnic background are considered as the basis for the establishment of quotas. These traits are considered important, particularly in studies of attitude and opinions. In nursing research, we can often include diagnosis and severity of illness as patient characteristics and occupational rank and educational preparation as characteristics of nurses.

The two examples used in this discussion of quota sampling both illustrated the case of two variables: the attitude of males and females toward the use of nurse practitioners, and the adequacy of preparation for labor based on the care provided by nurse midwives and physicians. The establishment of quotas for more than two variables is common. For example, a study of nursing students' preference for a career in nursing research might consider the present educational level and sex of the student. Quotas would need to be established for each sex and for each level of education such as freshmen, sophomores, juniors, and seniors. In this instance, quotas would be established for eight variables. The point to be emphasized is that the sample size must be large enough within each stratum to make possible an estimate of the population stratum. Generally, the more variables or characteristics that are used, the larger the sample size must be.

Quota sampling provides an improvement over accidental sampling but only when a conscientious effort is made to ensure that the sample contains diverse elements within the population. The selection of the cases to fill the quotas, however, is nonrandom; that is, those that happen to be available are selected. As with accidental sampling, there is no positive assurance that the cases selected within each quota fully represent the similarities and differences existing among the diverse elements of the target population.

Purposive sampling, the third nonprobability sampling procedure, involves handpicking the cases to be included in the sample. The procedure is founded on the belief that the investigator's knowledge about the population is sufficient to allow the selection of a sample judged to be representative of the target population. A basic assumption underlying purposive sampling is that the errors of judgment in the selection of the sample will tend to counterbalance each other. Experiments on purposive sampling suggest that without an objective basis for making the judgments, this is not a dependable assumption (Chein, 1976).

Although severely limiting in terms of generalizability of study findings, purposive samples are not uncommon. In the health field, studies of disease conditions are often based on such samples. For example, an investigator interested in a certain condition may select a sample from persons exhibiting symptoms of that condition. Depending upon the focus of the research, the purposive sample may be selected from the widest variety of cases or from those deemed to be average or representing the typical case. Purposive samples are also used to pretest newly developed instruments. In some instances, pretesting is based on a sample of divergent types of respondents, while in other cases, it is based on a homogeneous group of respondents known to hold some particular view or possess a certain trait.

SAMPLE SIZE

Determining the size of the sample is an important step in the process of sampling; but contrary to what the beginning researcher might expect, sample size estimation is really one of the last questions to be answered. It is also a very difficult and imprecise calculation. Various sample size formulas exist and can be found in a variety of statistical texts; however, because both approximation and guesswork are involved, application of the formulas requires more than the mathematical reduction of an equation. For interpretation and expression of the formulas, the interested reader might wish to consult Williams (1978) or Snedecor and Cochran (1967). For many research investigators, use of the formulas remains limited and unrealistic. First, the formulas are based on simple random sampling, and the opportunity to use that sampling procedure frequently does not arise. Second, research objectives usually include the study of many variables while the formulas are based on the events of one variable. Finally, the formulas are limited in their treatment of cost, and sample size generally can not be determined independent of the question of costs (Hess, Riedel, and Fitzpatrick, 1961).

Factors Influencing Sample Size

Several factors influence the size of samples. These include the dispersion of the target population, the degree of precision required, the risk specification, and the sampling procedure selected. Dispersion refers to the variability that exists within the defined target population. For example, if it is known that everyone attending an adolescent outpatient clinic is 13 years old, a sample of one would be sufficient to estimate their average age. The dispersion or variance in this example is zero, and one sampling element is all that is needed to estimate accurately the average age of the target population. More frequently researchers deal with populations that have variation, and their interest is in estimating from a sample the characteristics of the population. As a general rule, increasing sample size reduces the variance of the sample estimate.

Precision refers to how close the sample value should be to the true population value. Clearly there must be some statement of the precision required in a study. If it mattered little whether the sample estimate were near to or far from the true population value, then any sample size would be sufficient.

The curve of Figure 9-1 represents a rough approximation of the relationship between sample size and error (where error refers to deviation from population values). The figure illustrates that the smaller the sample, the larger will be the error, that is, the difference between the estimation of the population value and the true population value. This principle is not difficult to understand. The figures in Table 9-3 represent the ages of mothers in 10 random samples of two subjects each who received no anesthesia or analgesia during labor and delivery.

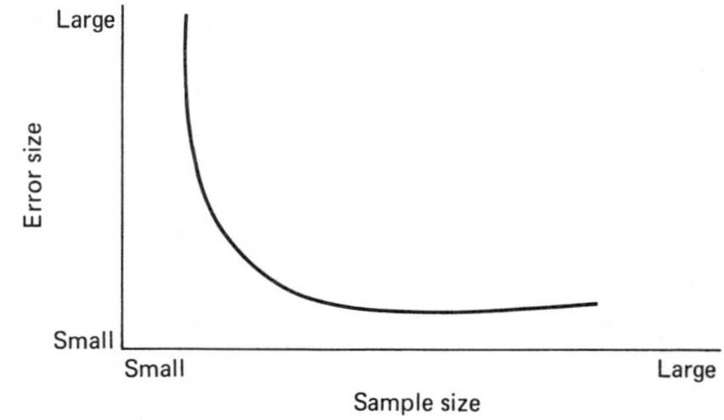

Figure 9-1. Relationship between sample size and sample error.

Table 9-3. Samples ($n = 2$) of Ages of Mothers at Time of Natural Childbirth Delivery

Age	19	33	16	21	17	13	16	15	19	22
Age	20	31	20	25	15	18	17	23	21	22
Mean	19.5	32	18	23	16	15.5	16.5	19	20	22
							Total mean for $n = 20 = 20.1$			

The means of the 10 samples diverge widely; the range is from 15.5 to 32, or 16.5 years. The mean of tbe target population of 115 mothers is 20.5 years with a range of 13 to 33, or 20 years. In practice, a researcher usually does not have the true population values to make this type of comparison. With very small samples like the ones illustrated in the table, researchers cannot have much confidence in their accuracy. Many of these samll samples do not provide good estimates of the true population value. When a sample size of 10 is selected by taking the first set of five samples from the table, the mean turns out to be 21.7 years. The mean of the second set of five samples turns out to be 18.6 years. The means of two other random samples of size $n = 10$ were 19.2 years and 22 years respectively. By increasing the sample size to $n = 10$, the variability has been reduced. Increasing the sample size to 20, using all of the samples in the table, results in an average age estimate of 20.1 years, which is very close to the true population value of 20.5 years. By now it should be clear that the difference between the sample estimate and the true population value can be reduced by increasing the size of the sample.

Closely associated with the question of precision or accuracy is the question of risk. Every sample is subject to the vagaries of random sampling; and, regardless of the precision specified, the actual sample value could turn out to be far from the true population value. For this reason a statement of the risk the researcher is willing to take needs to be made. For example, if the risk is established at 0.125, this means that of one sample in eight, the sample estimate will be farther away from the true population value than the specified precision. To reduce the risk, one generally must increase the sample size.

Finally, it has been mentioned that the type of sampling procedure selected has some impact on the question of sample size. This fact has been made evident in the preceding discussions of sampling procedures. For example, it was pointed out that for highly variable populations, stratified random sampling would be more efficient than simple random sampling. In general, variance can be reduced by carefully selecting sampling procedures that are appropriate to the natural grouping of the population. Although it was previously stated that increasing sample size has the desirable effect of reducing the sampling variance, it should be noted that the reduction diminishes progressively. The general rule is that to cut the variance in half, the sample size should be doubled. This is one of the reasons that the selection of an appropriate sampling procedure is so important. It can offer a much larger gain in terms of the efficiency of the study. An excellent discussion of the clever use of groups to reduce variance may be found in Williams (1978).

Practical Consideration

It should be evident from the foregoing discussion that determination of sample size proves to be a much less precise operation than a researcher might wish. Nevertheless, some general guidelines can be offered. The first is to select the best sampling procedure possible. The second is to take as large a sample as is economically and practically feasible. Although it is difficult to specify precisely what "large" is, some comments can be made on what it is not. It is generally agreed that samples of less than 10 are not sufficient. Moreover, the minimum of 10 refers to each of the subdivisions or cells of the data. If the study involves an experimental and control group, then a minimum of 10 respondents for each group is necessary for a total sample of $2 \times 10 = 20$. A study of the effects of a nursing procedure might require that respondents within each of the control and experimental groups be further subdivided according to sex (male and female) and age (65 and over, and under 65). In this instance, the sample size for both the experimental group and the control group would be $4 \times 10 = 40$, for a total sample of 80. Although a sample size of 10 can be considered a minimum, the researcher would be well advised to aim for a larger number, such as 20 or 30. Not only is the larger sample more likely to capture the true characteristics of the population, but also it prepares for the likely event that some respondents will refuse to participate in the investigation and some responses will prove to be of no value. The latter, of course, would be not because the responses are not in keeping with the hypothesis, but rather that they are incomprehensible or incomplete. In summary, then, the researcher should aim for a minimum sample size of 10, and preferably 20 or 30. The type of research study will dictate the need to plan for a larger sample to compensate for the possibility of nonresponse or incomplete response.

Before moving beyond the question of sample size, there is one more notion that needs to be discussed: the relationship between absolute sample size and relative sample size in a large population. As the population increases in size, the sample size required to obtain precise estimations remains fairly constant. In other words, the absolute size of the sample is more important than the sample size relative to population size. While a sample of 200, or 10%, may be necessary to obtain the required precision in estimating a population of 2,000, almost the same precision could be achieved with a sample size of 200, or 2%, of a population of 100,000. This is why, for example, samples of 1,000 or 2,000 are often sufficient to estimate certain characteristics of the entire United States population of over 200 million people. The notion that a 10% sample is four times as accurate as a 5% sample, or that a 20% sample is four times as accurate as a 5% sample, although seemingly plausible, is erroneous. Although it has been advised that as large a sample as possible should be obtained, when dealing with very large populations, expert counsel should be sought to avoid collecting wastefully large samples.

NONSAMPLING ERRORS

At the beginning of this chapter sampling errors were defined as the chance differences between the population estimate as obtained from a sample and the true population value. Differences of this nature can also be attributed to nonsampling errors, that is, factors other than those due to the process of sampling that can cause the sample to inaccurately represent the target population. They can be introduced in many ways and at various stages throughout a study. The major types of nonsampling errors include nonresponse errors, measurement errors, and data processing errors.

Nonresponse errors occur when a portion of the intended sample is excluded from analysis. This may happen for a variety of reasons: some people may refuse to answer the questionnaire or participate in the study, or interviewers do not follow their instructions or are unable to locate some of the intended respondents. For whatever reason, it is not uncommon that the intended sample is somewhat incomplete. The point to be emphasized is that it is generally unwise to assume that nonrespondents possess the same characteristics and to the same degree as the respondents. Although this is particularly evident in studies of sensitive issues, the question of the nonresponses should not be ignored even in studies of seemingly impersonal inquiry. Every effort should be made to reduce the number of nonresponses, and to the extent that they still occur, to describe them as thoroughly as possible. More will be said about this in the discussion of instruments in Chapter 10.

Measurement errors and data processing errors can be subtle and difficult to trace. All data collection, processing, and analysis procedures are subject to these types of errors, and their significance should not be underestimated. Nonsampling errors are often of greater magnitude than sampling errors. The larger the study, the harder it is to keep procedures under control, and thus the greater the chance for nonsampling errors to appear.

SUMMARY

In this chapter the importance and prevalence of sampling in research investigations have been discussed. Among the advantages of obtaining a sample rather than relying upon a complete census count is the fact that samples can often provide more accurate information. The definitions and concepts central to the understanding and application of sampling have been explained. These include the target population, subpopulation or population stratum, sampling element or population element, sampling unit, sampling frame, and sampling error. A clear and precise definition of the target population is the first and perhaps the most important step in the process of sampling.

Both probability and nonprobability sampling procedures have been defined along with the various approaches common to each. Probability sampling procedures employ the principles of random selection, whereas nonprobability sampling procedures rely on subjective decisions of the investigator. The distinction between the two types of procedures is particularly important to the identification of sampling error. Recall that some degree of sampling error is present in all samples regardless of the procedure used. When samples are selected through probability sampling procedures, an estimate of the magnitude of tbe sampling error can be made. There is, however, no way of estimating the extent of the sampling error with nonprobability sampling procedures. Simple random sampling, systematic sampling, stratified sampling, and cluster sampling are the probability sampling procedures desired by most research investigators. These procedures require the existence of a list or sampling frame of the population elements.

The selection of a particular probability sampling procedure or combination of procedures depends upon the circumstances of the research question. When probability samples are not possible, the investigator must select one of the nonprobability sampling procedures discussed: accidental sampling, quota sampling, or purposive sampling. When these procedures are employed, special care must be taken. There exists the potential for large sampling errors, and generalizability of findings is clearly restricted.

The question of sample size was discussed in detail by presenting the major factors that influence size, such as dispersion, precision, risk, and sampling procedure employed. Dispersion was defined as the variability of the population of interest. The greater the variability of the target population, the larger must be the sample size. Precision was discussed in terms of error, and again, larger samples tend to provide more precise sample estimates. It is up to the investigator to decide what level of precision is desirable or necessary. The notion of risk was also presented as a factor influencing sample size. Every time a sample is drawn there is a chance that it could be a very poor sample; that is, it would not closely approximate the characteristics of the population. The investigator must determine the amount of risk to be taken, and generally, the lower the risk, the larger the sample. Recognizing the complexity of sample size determination, it was advised that samples should not be smaller than 10, and more preferably should consist of 20 or 30 cases for each subdivision or cell of the data. Whenever possible, however, the investigator should consult with a statistician or expert in the field.

Finally, a short discussion of nonsampling errors was presented to remind the investigator that even when all efforts to select a sample truly representative of the population have been made, other potential errors can cause a disparity. The most common of these were defined as nonresponse errors, measurement errors, and data processing errors.

BIBLIOGRAPHY

Babbie, E.R. *Survey Research Methods.* Belmont: Wadsworth, 1973, pp. 73–108.

Chein, I. An introduction to sampling, in Selltiz, C., Wrightsman, L.S., and Cook, S.W. (Eds.), *Research Methods in Social Relations,* 3rd Edition. New York: Holt, Rinehart and Winston, 1976, pp. 512–540.

Hess, I., Riedel, D.C., & Fitzpatrick, T.B. *Probability Sampling of Hospitals and Patients.* Bureau of Hospital Administration, Research Series No. 1. Ann Arbor: The University of Michigan, 1961.

Snedecor, G.W., & Cochran, W.G. *Statistical Methods,* 6th edition. Ames, Iowa: The Iowa State University Press, 1967.

Warwick, D.P., & Lininger, C.A. *The Sample Survey: Theory and Practice.* New York: McGraw-Hill, 1975, pp. 72–73.

Williams, B. *A Sampler on Sampling.* New York: John Wiley & Sons, 1978.

10
Instruments for Data Collection

Sandra J. Eyres

Planning a study is a decision-making process. No matter how complex or simple the study, decisions have to be made about the conceptual approach that will be used, the specific purpose or purposes of the study, and the way in which data will be obtained to serve the purpose of the study. One of the major decisions to be made, the focus of this chapter, is the method of data production; the findings will be no stronger than this link in the chain of decision.

DATA PRODUCTION

Data production refers to how information from the real world can be elicited, systematically recorded, and quantified. Different methods of data production can have different ways of eliciting, recording, and quantifying information. It is helpful to think of these parts of the data production process separately in trying to understand the utility of different data collection instruments. Data collection instruments are the tools used in the data production process. These tools or instruments may assist with all three portions of data production; eliciting, recording, and quantifying. On the other hand, a specific instrument might serve only as a way of recording and quantifying or as a way either to record or to quantify information. This will become clearer with some examples as in Table 10-1. The examples are all for typical variables in studies of child health and development, and they show some of the diversity of data production methods even within a single field of study.

Social status is a variable often used in nursing research. Socioeconomic indicators of life-style are associated with many aspects of health,

Table 10-1. Examples of Data Production

Variable	*Possible Sources*	*Methods of Eliciting*	*Methods of Recording*	*Methods of Quantifying*
Social status	Existing records	Review records	Devised form	Hollingshead Two Factor Index (1957)
	Subject	Questionnnaire	Questionnaire	Hollingshead Two Factor Index (1957)
Gestational age	Mother	Medical history	Medical record	Formula based on date of last menstrual period
	Newborn	Physical examination	Special form	Scoring system by Dubowitz, et al. (1970)
Mother's attentiveness	Mother	Interview	Interview recording form	Quantity as reported
	Mother-child interaction	Ask mother to teach child	Observer rates behavior on form	The rating assigned by the observer
	Mother-child interaction	Ask mother to teach child	Video tape	Computerized counting system

such as exposure to stressful conditions, ability to obtain health care, beliefs about illness, and health-related behavior. There are a variety of ways to produce data on socioeconomic status. Sometimes the information already exists in records. Eliciting it, after getting the necessary permission, is a matter then of reviewing the records. The form used on which to record the variables, designed specifically for that purpose, can be thought of as the instrument. From this recorded information the variable social status could then be quantified or numerically represented using a method devised by Hollingshead (1957). There are many different methods of quantifying socioeconomic status; this particular one combines assigned weights for occupation and education.

A more frequently used method of eliciting information on socioeconomic status is to ask the study participants, since the participants are likely to have the most accurate and latest information on their occupation, educational background, and marital status. The asking can be done verbally (interview) or in writing (questionnaire). As in our example, when a questionnaire is used, it is the instrument and serves both the eliciting and recording functions. Again, if the Hollingshead index is used to quantify socioeconomic status, these calculations are done using the information from the instrument.

In the second example in Table 10-1, the variable is gestational age. The traditional means of eliciting this information is to ask mothers the date of their last menstrual period. This is usually done verbally as part of the medical history, and the estimated date of conception becomes part of the medical record. Gestational age can then be quantified by comparing the expected to the actual time of the birth. Here, except for a medical record abstracting form, instrumentation plays a minor part in producing data.

In recent years another method of determining gestational age was devised by Dubowitz, Dubowitz, and Goldberg (1970). This method uses the newborn, rather than the mother, as the source of information. Obviously the information cannot be elicited by asking; instead, information is obtained by examining babies directly. Following a prescribed procedure, the examiner looks for neurologic and other physical signs and records the findings on a specially designed form that facilitates calculations for individual babies to determine their gestational age. In this instance the data collection instrument is the recording form and also the scoring system, which clearly describes the signs to look for and gives instructions as to how to calculate the estimated gestational age.

So far factual information, such as education and occupation, and physical data, such as gestational age, have been discussed. There are other basic types of information often sought in nursing research. In the third example in Table 10-1, the variable of interest is the mother's attentiveness to the child's cues of distress or the need for help. Here the interest is in how mothers respond, that is, their behavior.

A variety of methods can be used to produce data about behavior. One of the simplest is to ask what people do. In the example the mother could be given a questionnaire in which she is asked how long she lets the baby cry before going to see what's wrong. Her report of the number of minutes could be accepted as the quantified variable.

Sometimes, however, what people say they do does not coincide with what they actually do owing to inaccurate memory or recall of what they typically do and a hesitancy to give answers that may be socially frowned upon. For example, mothers are unlikely to watch a clock to time how long they wait before going to a crying baby. And, if their tendency is to wait for what seems to them a long time, they may report a shorter time to avoid being considered insensitive and cruel.

For these reasons investigators often prefer to elicit data on behavior by direct observation. The mother could be asked to teach her child a task. An observer could then watch the mother's and child's behavior and record ratings of the observed cues and attentiveness on an instrument.

If investigators doing a study of mothers' attentive behavior wanted to be even more objective and precise in producing the data, they might choose more complicated instruments. Instruments also can be mechanical devices. The sessions of mothers teaching their children could be videotaped. The recordings from this mechanical instrument could then be observed and quantified using yet other instruments; while watching the videotapes observers could manually enter specific defined activities, movements, or positions into a computerized system designed for behavioral research. The computer then would do the quantifying.

Many other mechanical instruments are used as measurement tools in nursing research. They range from relatively simple devices, such as a thermometer, to more complex ones, such as the application of telemetry in monitoring physiological events. The focus of this chapter is mainly on nonmechanical instruments, but the reader should be aware of mechanical instruments and the important role they play in nursing research. Further information can be found in books devoted to this topic (Geddes and Baker, 1968; Johnson and Lubin, 1972; and Cromwell, et al., 1976).

The examples in Table 10-1 illustrate that there are multiple ways to produce data and different procedures use different types of instruments to elicit, record, or quantify data. Now consider some specific types of data collection instruments and the different ways they elicit, record, and quantify information.

DATA COLLECTION INSTRUMENTS

Questionnaire

Questionnaires are a pencil-and-paper method of asking respondents for information. A questionnaire can contain questions asked in a variety of formats. For example, the question might give several alternatives from which the respondent is asked to check the most appropriate one: these are called multiple choice questions. A check-off list can also be used for which the respondent is asked to check those alternatives which apply. Or open-ended questions can be used that provide space for the respondent to write in the answers in sentences or phrases. Questionnaires and how to construct them are discussed more fully in Chapter 11. Figure 10-1 shows items from a typical questionnaire designed to produce demographic data.

There are several advantages to questionnaires. They are usually the simplest, quickest, and least expensive way to collect data. The respondents can read the questions for themselves and record the answers directly on the form. Questionnaires do not necessarily require the presence of the investigator; other people at the locale can distribute them to subjects and collect them upon completion. For instance, if a study involved out-patients and the symptoms they had experienced since the last visit, those people who routinely receive patients for their clinic visit could distribute the questionnaires about symptoms and collect them after the patients had completed them. This type of procedure, of course, requires special arrangements within the care setting; permission of those involved must be obtained and a way must be found to protect the confidentiality of the responses on the completed questionnaires.

Questionnaires can also be used without any person-to-person contact. If addresses for persons in the sample are known, questionnaires can be mailed to the subjects with the request that answers be returned by enclosed stamped preaddressed envelopes. Typically, the response rate for mailed questionnaires, however, is lower than for those distributed in person. The personal touch can be an added incentive to complete a questionnaire.

The absence of the investigator during completion of a questionnaire can be one of the main disadvantages of this method of data collection.

1. How old are you?

   ______years old

2. What do you consider to be your ethnic background?

   ______Caucasian

   (1)

   ______Afro-American/Black

   (2)

   ______Chicano/Mexican-American

   (3)

   ______Asian

   (4)

   ______American Indian

   (5)

   ______Other (please specify)________________________________

   (6)

3. What is your occupation? ________________________________

   ____

4. Have you done this work for pay during the past year?

   ______No

   (0)

   ______Yes

   (1)

5. Do you receive your major support from public assistance?

   ______No

   (0)

   ______Yes

   (1)

6. What is your total family income per month?

   Amount per month ______

7. How many years of schooling have you completed?

   ______Number of years of schooling

8. What is the *highest* degree you have obtained?

   ______High School

   (1)

   ______College (undergraduate)

   (2)

Figure 10-1. Example of questionnaire items.

_____Trade or vocational
(3)
_____Graduate (Masters, Ph.D.)
(4)

9. What is your present marital status?

_____Married (1)	_____Never married (5)
_____Divorced (2)	_____Common-law (6)
_____Separated (3)	_____Living together (7)
_____Widowed (4)	_____Other (please specify): (8) ____________

Figure 10-1. *(Continued)*

Respondents cannot clarify questions or terms which may be unclear to them. Nevertheless, the questionnaire is probably the most frequently used instrument in research because it takes less time and resources to produce data than other types of instruments do.

Interview

The interview method of data collection is essentially the same as a questionnaire except that the interviewer verbally asks questions of the respondent. The term "interview" often is used on radio and television. Research interviews differ from those on the news media in that the former aim systematically to elicit the same information from all subjects. This means that the same questions are asked in as similar a manner as possible. The instrument in this case is called the interview schedule, the list of questions to be asked. The interviewer records the responses directly on the interview schedule or on an accompanying form. Figure 10-2 is a portion of an interview schedule. This interview was used in an exploratory study of the problems of families with terminally ill children (Williams, 1979).

One of the major advantages of the interview is the presence of the interviewer, who can clarify questions that are not clear. Interviewers can also use probes (additional prompting questions) if the subject provides little information or seems hesitant. If probes are used, they

1. How severely have your daily routines been disrupted since ______'s illness?

   a. During the time when a child is sick, many parents find it difficult to complete household tasks. Do you find that this is a problem for you?

      Yes______. No______.

      (If answer is yes, go to 1b. If answer is no, proceed to number 2)

   b. Who do you have to help you with the household tasks?

2. Who do you turn to for help in caring for your children?

   a. How often do you need additional help?

3. What changes, if any, have you noticed in how you spend your free time?

   a. Do you see your friends more or less often than before ______was sick? More time______. Less Time______.

   b. Do you feel that now you have less in common with your friends? Yes______. No______.

      (If answer is yes, proceed to 3b1. If answer is no, proceed to number 4)

      1. Would you like to comment on that?

4. How have family responsibilities changed since your child has become ill?

   a. Who is the person that is with ______ the most amount of time?

Figure 10-2. Example of interview schedule. (From Williams, H.A., *Perceived Needs and Support Systems of Single Parents with Children Diagnosed with a Life-Threatening Illness,* unpublished Master's thesis, University of Washington, 1979. Reprinted with permission of Holly A. Williams.)

should be part of the interview schedule so that they, along with the basic questions, are the same for all subjects.

In the interview form of instrumentation, there is a human factor in eliciting and recording the information. While this can be an advantage in obtaining more and clearer data, care is needed in planning the study so that, if multiple interviewers are involved, differences in their behavior will not confound the data. Before conducting the study, a period of training is helpful so that the interviewers become familiar with the procedures. Possible questions should be asked in a similar manner so that the information solicited is comparable for all subjects.

There are many ways, some subtle and some not so subtle, in which interviewers can vary in the information they elicit. Barath and Cannell (1977), for example, became aware of differences in interviewers' voice intonation. To obtain information on people's health, the interviewers read from a checklist of symptoms and conditions and marked those that the subjects reported experiencing. At the end of each symptom or condition from the checklist some interviewers lowered their voices and others raised their voices so that the reading of the item sounded more like a question. Using an experimental design, they tested whether these different intonations produced different responses from the subjects. They found that subjects reported significantly more symptoms and conditions when the interviewers used the rising intonation as in questioning.

Even if only one interviewer does all the interviews for a study, some differences in information can result by changes over time in how the interviewer asks questions. The individual interviewer should try to be as consistent as possible over the course of the study.

A pretest of the interview instrument is invaluable in deciding how questions should be asked. For example, Holly Williams (personal communication, 1979), who devised the interview from which the example items were taken in Fig. 10-2, found that parents provided much more information when the word "comfort" was verbally emphasized in this item: When (child's name) is in the hospital, do you feel *comfort*able leaving him? The emphasis placed by the interviewer can elicit different thought processes than would otherwise be the case.

Another potential problem with interviews is the process of recording responses. Verbatim recording of verbal responses is tedious and time consuming. Some of the accuracy or completeness of responses can be lost in the process. Also, the emotion expressed by the respondents in the way they said their responses cannot be captured in the written recording. To overcome these potential problems, investigators sometimes record the interviews on an audio tape recorder. This method of recording helps to ensure both the accuracy of the record of the verbal response and the affect with which it was given. This procedure, like all aspects of data collection, must be weighed both for its advantages and disadvantages: some subjects might be more reticent to talk with a tape recorder going or might unconsciously modify the intensity of their responses.

All in all, however, the interview is a very valuable technique in nursing research. It is especially useful in exploratory studies, in studies where the information sought is not of a simple factual nature, and in studies where eliciting the data in person is desirable for completeness of information. Further information on interview instruments and interviewing technique is available in other published material (Connell and Kahn, 1968; Meadow and Gass, 1963; Selltiz, et al., 1976).

Instruments for Measuring Opinions

For the most part questionnaires and interviews are used to obtain factual information. Nursing researchers are also interested in another broad type of information: people's opinions. The term opinion is used here to cover a wide range of terminology present in the literature, such as attitudes, perceptions, expectations, and so on. There are many types of instruments used to measure opinions. The majority have been developed in the disciplines of psychology, sociology, and education.

Rating

One of the basic principles used in instruments to measure opinion variables is rating. Rating means to assign a numerical value somewhere on a defined continuum. Grading students and clinical proficiency reports are common forms of rating.

In research the subjects may be asked to rate other people on certain qualities, or they may be asked to do self-rating. Also, subjects can be asked to rate objects, events, or circumstances to obtain a measure of their perceptions.

A rating in which a single question or item is used is referred to as an indice or indicator. An index has been created if two or more indicators are used to rate according to some defined procedure. The Hollingshead Index of Social Class (1957) mentioned earlier is a good example. Individuals are assigned separate numerical ratings for occupation and education. These are combined into an index of social class.

Scaling

Scaling is another term for rating using multiple indicators: this refers to a meaningful way of combining ratings among items to assign an overall numerical value. Instruments using this technique are referred to as scales. For example, if we wanted to study patients' perceptions of their upcoming surgery, we might ask the following:

Do you think you will recover quickly from your operation?

☐ *No* ☐ *Undecided* ☐ *Yes*

Patients' answers to this indicator would allow us to assign a numerical rating: No = 1, Undecided = 2, Yes = 3. But this gross way of measuring the variable "perception of surgery" has some weaknesses. First of all, the item taps only a portion of what patients may anticipate about surgery; there are certainly many thoughts that preoccupy people before they undergo an operation. If there were more items, we could learn more about the patients' opinions about the upcoming experience and, therefore, would have a stronger measure of the variable. Another way of stating this is that, with more items, the measure of the patients' perceptions would be more reliable. It is desirable for a scale to have at least 8 to 10 items (Smith, 1975).

The alternatives for responding to the hypothetical example are also too limited. They would not reflect the variability that is likely to exist in presurgical patients' opinions. Respondents are likely to have finer gradations of perceptions on either side of "undecided" than are shown by checking only "yes" or "no." The example also violates the tradition in attitude measurement that items should be statements rather than questions (Edwards, 1957). This is because questions imply knowledge and facts, and people are more likely to answer questions based on what is socially acceptable.

Now let us look at an example that overcomes these deficiencies. Palmer (1965) developed an instrument called the Patient's Perception Scale that measures the adult patient's perception of impending general surgery. Figure 10-3 shows several of the 46 statements contained in the scale. This scale gives the patient five alternative responses to each item from "strongly agree" to "strongly disagree." The statements in the total scale were chosen to cover several categories of perceptions including confidence in the ability of the family to maintain itself; skill and competence of physician, hopsital, and staff; body integrity; and acceptance of the need for surgery.

This instrument is an example of a Likert-type scale. On this type of scale the number of responses generally allowed is five. Scores are assigned from five (for strongly agree) to one (for strongly disagree). The scores are then added for all the items to get a total score or rating for the individual patient. Scales that use this form of scoring are called summated rating scales.

Another scaling method is the semantic differential technique. This technique was developed by Snider and Osgood (1969) and measures concepts by their position in "semantic space." Adjectives are used to anchor the continua or scales, and respondents are asked to mark the position along the scales that best reflects their view of the concept. The spaces along the scale are assigned numerical values; there is a variety of methods for combining and anlyzing scores for the scales (Kerlinger,

1. Soon I am going to be able to do all the things I used to do.
   Strongly agree________, Agree________, Undecided________, Disagree________, Strongly disagree________.
2. The people who are closest to me in my family can take this in their stride.
   Strongly agree________, Agree________, Undecided________, Disagree________, Strongly disagree________.
3. I can be up and doing things for myself in a few days.
   Strongly agree________, Agree________, Undecided________, Disagree________, Strongly disagree________.
4. Surgery is a quick way to get well.
   Strongly agree________, Agree________, Undecided________, Disagree________, Strongly disagree________.
5. Surgery is much safer today than it was in my parents' time.
   Strongly agree________, Agree________, Undecided________, Disagree________, Strongly disagree________.
6. The staff help make people comfortable when they have pain.
   Strongly agree________, Agree________, Undecided________, Disagree________, Strongly disagree________.

Figure 10-3. Example of Likert-type scale items. (Reprinted with permission of Irene S. Palmer. The development of a measuring device: Measuring patients' perceptions toward impending surgery, *Nursing Research*, 1965, 14:100–105.)

1973, pp. 566–581). Figure 10-4 shows items from the Semantic Differential for Health (SDH), an application of the basic technique by Jenkins (1966). The total SDH contains 16 items, and each item is referred to as a separate scale. This instrument was used to study beliefs about the concepts of tuberculosis, poliomyelitis, cancer, and mental illness.

Rating scales are useful research tools. They are a relatively efficient way to elicit, record, and quantify information about attitudes and opinions. Respondents often find them interesting to complete, and they are easy to administer. As with any type of data collection instrument they also have potential difficulties.

One potential problem with rating scales is referred to by Kerlinger (1973) as an extrinsic weakness. This is the tendency for people to use existing scales indiscriminantly. Not all scales, even if designed to measure the same variable, are of equal quality. The process of developing a valid, reliable scale is a rigorous one requiring time, empirical testing, and application of psychometric techniques (Anastasi, 1968).

Other potential problems with rating scales center around systematic response biases. Bias due to social desirability has already been mentioned. Rating scales are not necessarily free from this type of bias, especially if it is evident to the respondent what the scale is meant to measure.

Other types of response bias have to do with the tendency to rate items similarly. Respondents may avoid using the extreme values, that is, the lowest and highest ratings. Or they may rate all items high or low. The tendency to agree with items regardless of their content is called acquiescent response set (Batey, 1979). To avoid this, items are sometimes alternated in their wording so the high rating is not always equivalent to a positive response. The following hypothetical items which might appear on a scale to measure depression illustrate this:

I have trouble sleeping.

☐ *Never* ☐ *Seldom* ☐ *Occasionally* ☐ *Frequently* ☐ *Almost always*

I feel a sense of accomplishment after a day's work.

☐ *Never* ☐ *Seldom* ☐ *Occasionally* ☐ *Frequently* ☐ *Almost always*

If item reversal is done, then, of course, consideration must be given to the positive or negative nature of the statement when scores are summed among items. For the example items, to derive a total depres-

A.	Many people get it		Some people get it		A few people get it	Almost nobody gets it
B.	This is usually a disease of					
	Babies	Children	Teenagers	Young adults	Middle age	Very old people
C.	Is extremely painful		Causes much pain	Causes some pain	Causes little pain but is uncomfortable	Causes very little discomfort
D.	People recover fully		People recover but are weaker		People have permanent minor body damage	People have obvious permanent disability
E.	Usually causes death		Often causes death		Sometimes causes death	Rarely causes death
F.	Clean		Sort of clean		Sort of dirty	Dirty

Figure 10-4. Examples of semantic differential items. (From Jenkins, C.D., The semantic differential for health: A technique for measuring beliefs about diseases, *Public Health Reports*, June 1966, *81*, pp. 549–558. Reprinted with permission of C. David Jenkins.)

sion score the respondent would be assigned a 5 for the first item if the fifth alternative were checked and another 5 if the first alternative were checked on the second item. That is, scores are assigned in reverse for the positively stated items.

Other Applications of Instruments

Unlike those for opinions, attitudes, and beliefs, instruments developed to measure knowledge are based on the assumption that there is a correct answer. Therefore, items are usually in the form of questions, and scores are assigned according to the number of correct responses. Students in nursing, as in any other discipline, are very familiar with tests of their knowledge. This type of instrument has become more frequently used in health-related research as interest in health education, prevention, and self-care have increased.

Figure 10-5 shows some items from an instrument developed by

Sex Knowledge Test (Form A)

1. Where do babies come from?
   a. from the hospital
   b. out of the mother
   c. from some place else
2. How often do most women menstruate?
   a. once a week
   b. once a month
   c. once a year
3. When does a new baby begin to grow?
   a. when the mother releases an egg
   b. when the father releases a sperm
   c. when the sperm meets the egg
4. Why do some people use birth control?
   a. because they want to have a baby
   b. because they don't want to have a baby right then
   c. because they want twins
5. A woman can become pregnant only:
   a. if she is married
   b. if she is in love
   c. if she has intercourse

Figure 10-5. Example items from a knowledge test. (Reprinted with permission of Doris Bloch, *Attitudes and Practices of Mothers in the Sex Education of Their Daughters*. Unpublished doctoral dissertation, University of California, Berkeley, 1970.)

Bloch (1970) that elicit information on sex knowledge. There is one alternative from each item that is correct. The number of correct answers is divided by 25, since this is the total number of items. The result is then multiplied by 100 to get a percentage score for the individual respondent. This is an example of the use of multiple choice items.

Skill and ability can also be measured by observing performance. For

Behaviors Evaluated	Satisfactory	Unsatisfactory
I. Assumes professional responsibility		
A. Professional behavior		
1. Hair arranged so as not to contaminate working area		
2. Patient information treated with confidentiality		
3. Avoids discussing personal life in clinical area		
4. Prepared to begin care on unit at correct time		
5. Addresses resident/client by preferred title		
6. Protects resident/client's privacy while administering care		
II. Communications		
A. Interaction		
1. Verbally communicates with resident		
2. Nonverbally communicates with resident		
3. Explains procedures		
4. Does patient teaching		
B. Written communication		
Without assistance correctly charts:		
1. On nurse's notes:		
a. subjective data		
b. objective data		
c. analysis		
d. plan		

Figure 10-6. Example items from a performance test. (From *N281 Clinical Evaluation Tool*. Reprinted with permission of Anne Lousteau.)

example, Loustau (in press) and her teaching colleagues have developed an instrument to evaluate the clinical performance of nursing students. Figure 10-6 shows a few of the items from this tool. This instrument is an example of a checklist format. The number of items checked satisfactory can be used as a score. Reliability is a major potential problem when observational methods of measurement are used. Realizing this, Loustau and her colleagues used videotapes of students' performance to test interrater reliability. Rating from videotapes is a very useful method for testing this type of reliability on observational tools. When disagreements on ratings occur, this method helps identify problematic items, unclear wording, or the need for clearer instructions.

Interrater reliability was tested in the same manner for the instrument shown in part in Figure 10-7 (Barnard and Eyres, 1979). This is also an

---

Maternal Behavior

A. Contingent Positive Feedback (Verbal and Nonverbal)

Positive feedback here is defined as either verbal (e.g., "Good for you," "That's right," etc.) or nonverbal (patting, hugging, smiling at infant) behavior which is clearly approving of something the infant has just done which is compatible with the teaching process.

0. Not applicable. Infant never did anything appropriate (i.e., never attended, never attempted, etc.).
1. Never. Mother gave no positive feedback.
2. Once or twice.
3. Occasionally: 3–5times.
4. Frequently: 6+ times.
5. Continuous positive feedback given to infant's task-appropriate behavior.

B. Contingent Negative Feedback (Verbal and Nonverbal)

Mother's negative feedback, either verbal (e.g., "No," "That's wrong," "Don't do that") or nonverbal (slapping, spanking, taking infant's hand or materials from mouth, taking materials from infant's hands, etc.) follows infant's task-inappropriate behavior, including inattention.

Figure 10-7. Example scales for rating behavior. (Reprinted with permission of Kathryn E. Barnard & Sandra J. Eyres [Eds.], *Child Health Assessment Part 2: The First Year of Life*, U.S. Department of Health, Education, and Welfare, Health Resources Administration, Division of Nursing, DHEW Publication No. HRA 79-25, 1979.) *(Continued on page 208.)*

Even though some mothers may "correct" and reprimand in a playful manner, the reprimand should be rated as negative feedback because of the content. Note that inhibiting the infant's behavior is considered negative feedback.

0. Not applicable. Infant did nothing inappropriate or incompatible with task performance.
1. Never.
2. Once or twice.
3. Occasionally: 3–5 times.
4. Frequently: 6+ times.
5. Continuous negative feedback for task-incompatible behavior. Infant is unable to get away with anything.

C. Modeling

Mother demonstrates or models all or part of task (i.e., she shows him all or part of what she wants him to do).

1. Never.
2. Once.
3. Occasionally: 2–5 times.
4. Frequently: 6+ times.
5. Nearly constantly. Infant can hardly do the task due to mother's possession of the materials.

Figure 10-7. *(Continued)*

observational tool and is an example of how rating scales can be used in measuring behavior. In this instance, the instrument was designed to score the mother's behavior after she teaches her child an age-specific task. For further information on behavioral observation, see Sackett (1978), Byerly (1976), Hutt and Hutt (1970), Pascall and Jenkins (1961), and Weick (1968).

The examples in this chapter illustrate some of the diversity of data collection instruments. They can elicit information by asking subjects for facts or judgments. The information can be recorded in a variety of formats including checklists and multiple-choice or more complicated scales. The format can serve as the method of quantifying the information, as in scales, or the investigator can translate the information into numerical values using a formula external to the instrument.

CHOOSING A DATA COLLECTION INSTRUMENT

How does an investigator decide what collection instrument to use? This decision will be influenced by several factors:

1. The purpose of the study. Some types of instruments will probably serve the study purpose better than others. As has been discussed, different types of instruments produce different types of information. Questions, as on questionnaires and interview schedules, generate information of a factual nature or test respondent's knowledge. Statements, as on rating scales, call for opinion or judgment.
2. The validity of the instrument. Validity is a central issue in choosing instruments, that is, how well does it measure what you want to measure? As discussed in Chapter 8, there are different types of validity. Instruments that have had extensive use are more likely to have been tested for these different types of validity. For others the investigator in search of an instrument might find no report of validity.
3. The reliability of the instrument. As explained in Chapter 8, reliability refers to "will the same methods used by different researchers and/or at different times produce the same results?" (Smith, 1975, p. 58). As with validity, the reports of tests for reliability will vary. If different instruments are available to measure the same variable, choosing one with high reported validity and reliability will help to ensure the quality of the data produced.
4. The feasibility of using the instrument. Instruments vary in their ease of application. Some require more time, money, and personnel than others; if resources are limited, this can play an important part in the choice of instruments.
5. The instructions for the instrument. If respondents are unclear as to what they are expected to do, the validity and reliability of the instrument are jeopardized. To the researcher, checklists or fill-in-the-blank questions look simple. Care should be taken that they appear equally simple and clear to the subjects. Investigators usually clarify the instructions with a verbal or written explanation for the respondent at the beginning of the instrument or at steps in the data collection contact where the format of the instrument changes.
6. The language of the instrument. There is a tendency to forget that some people cannot read at all and that others may not be familiar with the esoteric terminology used by investigators steeped in a particular topic of interest. The validity of an instrument is strengthened if the language in it is understandable to all and if interviews are used for potentially illiterate subjects.
7. The time required by the respondent to complete the instrument. Instruments vary in the length of time required to complete them. There is a fatigue factor in being a subject in a study. This is

especially true if two or more instruments are used in combination for the same data collection contact. The attention of the subject decreases after one or one-and-a-half hours of responding to questions and making judgments about statements. Thus, there is some advantage in choosing the shortest way to measure any one variable in a study. The time required is often important in health-related studies since the subjects may have health problems that make them particularly vulnerable to fatigue.

8. Previous use of the instrument. It is often highly desirable to be able to compare the study findings with those of other investigators who have studied the same topic. These comparisons are greatly facilitated if the same instrumentation is used.

Evaluating instruments for their pros and cons helps in choosing a specific instrument. In reality it is often the case that none of the alternative instruments is perfect on all of the above points. The investigator then has the option of deciding which attributes are most important for a particular study and making the best choice possible realizing the limitations.

FINDING DATA COLLECTION INSTRUMENTS

How does one go about finding alternative data collection instruments from which to choose? This is often one of the results of the literature review done for a study. In reports of studies on the topic in which the investigator is interested, other investigators will explain the instruments they used and give the sources where the instruments can be located. This is one of the best ways of locating instruments, especially if one wants to compare findings with those of past studies.

One can also locate instruments by communicating with investigators who have a study in progress or have completed research on the topic of interest. Usually people who do research are quite willing to talk with others by letter or telephone to give advice and share their experience with specific instruments.

In planning a study there is no substitute for discussing ideas with those who are knowledgeable. These discussions not only alert us to potential pitfalls in our design, but they can also prompt specific suggestions including some on instrumentation.

There are numerous published compilations of instruments for different areas of measurement (Buros, 1978; Comrey, 1973; Goldman, 1974; Johnson and Bommarito, 1971; Robinson and Shaver, 1973;

Robinson, Rusk, and Head, 1968; Robinson, Athansiou, and Head, 1969; Strauss, 1969). Some compilations are specific to instruments used in nursing research (Ward and Lindeman, 1978; Ward and Fetler, 1979). Many compilations are helpful because, in addition to the instrument itself, they contain a review and evaluation of the instrument. They summarize the reports of validity, reliability, and other aspects to be taken into consideration when choosing an instrument.

WHEN ALTERNATIVES DO NOT EXIST

Sometimes, no matter how hard one looks, existing instruments cannot be found to measure the study variables. Then there is little option but to develop a tool for data collection. Depending on the complexity of the information, this can be time consuming and requires knowledge of the principles of instrument construction. It is rare, however, that existing instruments will be found to collect all of the information for a study. Usually some questionnaire or interview items are needed to measure the mediating or confounding variables which are specific to the study. Developing such instruments is discussed in Chapter 11.

While developing instruments from scratch can be an awesome undertaking, caution is healthy before accepting an available tool too readily. An instrument should serve the investigator rather than vice versa. A tool can be highly valid and reliable, but that is irrelevant if it does not measure the specific variables of interest.

AIDS IN USING DATA COLLECTION INSTRUMENTS

Consultation from a statistician can be very helpful in recognizing the level of measurement possible with different instrument formats. (Level of measurement was discussed in Chapter 8.) Statisticians can also help determine the appropriate analytic methods to be used. Their help should be sought early in the planning process rather than after the data are collected. Their advice can beneficially influence the development of and form of instrumentation used to collect the data.

When possible, a pretest of the data production process is always advantageous. A pretest is a trial prior to the full study; it is an opportunity to find out what works and what doesn't work so that necessary changes can be made before the study. The pretest trial can show whether respondents understand the instructions, whether the items are clear, whether they produce the type of information desired, and whether the overall data production process is feasible. If a large enough number of subjects is included in the pretest, tests of reliability can also be done. The value of the pretest is enhanced if the subjects are similar to those who will be in the subsequent study but are not the same individuals. If the same individuals responded to both the pretest and the full study instruments, the pretest experience with the instruments could influence how they respond later in the study.

Although the invitation to participate in the study and the explanation of the value of the research are technically not part of the data collection instrument, the manner in which these explanations are delivered can affect the success of applying the instrument. This is especially true if the instrument appears complicated or time consuming. The chance of gaining participation is enhanced if the invitation shows respect for the respondent, and if the explanation is logically convincing about the value of the subject's investment of time. In developing these precursors of data collection and the actual items on the instrument, it is helpful to put oneself in the role of the potential respondent. If a complete stranger approached you with the communications of the data collection process that you have developed, how would you react? Colleagues who are more objective about your study can also be helpful in evaluating the impression your communications make.

The appearance of instruments can also influence their chance of successfully eliciting information. Messy or hard-to-read forms are very uninviting. They give the general impression that the investigator is not capable or does not place enough value on the research to put the time and resources into developing an efficient instrument.

Sometimes investigators have no choice about the setting in which instruments are administered: it may be dictated by the purpose of the research, for example, describing nurses' activities in intensive care units. In other instances the setting should be chosen to enhance the quality of the data produced. Privacy during an interview might encourage subjects to be more open in their responses. The quietness and comfort of the setting can foster more attention to the task at hand and, therefore, increase the validity of the data.

FURTHER COMMENTS ON THE DATA PRODUCTION PROCESS

This chapter began by considering the different components of data production. It concluded by trying to put data collection instruments into perspective in relation to this overall process. Instruments are the tools used in data production, but the process is broader than the tools used as examples here.

There are many techniques for eliciting data. Besides asking subjects for responses, there are many variations on the observational technique, such as direct, participant, and nonparticipant observation. There are also projective techniques in which data are elicited through such methods as showing pictures or participating in psychodrama. Or data may have been elicited in the past, and existing records can be used as the source. Depending on the technique for eliciting data, the instrument can play a major or minor role in this part of the data production process. Therefore, before deciding on instrumentation, the investigator must be clear on the basic technique most desirable for eliciting data.

Instruments play an important part in recording information. They serve as the permanent record of the raw data (the form of the data elicited before any transformations are done for analysis). As was seen, these records can take many forms, ranging from a checklist, open-ended questions, to a highly structured rating scale (Oppenheim, 1966, Chap. 4). They can also be relatively blank sheets on which relatively unstructured information is recorded. The form of the instrument as a recording device will depend on the technique used to elicit data and the type of quantification to be done.

The quantification part of the data production process can also vary beyond the assigning of numerical values, which has been stressed in the examples used in this chapter. Responses can be analyzed for categories of communication they contain, as in content analysis (Holsti, 1968). They might also be used to classify individuals into qualitative categories (Selltiz, et al., 1974, pp. 460–473). Or they may be examined for the essence of meaning, as in exploratory studies that are done to help construct quantifiable variables. To reiterate, the quantification or analytic portion of the data production process will influence the form of instrumentation.

SUMMARY

In summary, there are many considerations in selecting and using data collection instruments, some of the most important of which are the compatibilities or incompatibilities of the instruments with the overall data production process. This chapter has presented the information needed for the use of questionnaires and introductions as well as tools to measure opinions and knowledge. Also presented were methods for using rating and scaling. Other considerations included the qualities, such as validity, reliability, and feasibility, of specific tools. The reader is given relevant examples and references for additional readings throughout the chapter.

BIBLIOGRAPHY

Anastasi, A. *Psychological Testing,* 3rd edition. New York: Macmillan, 1968.

Barath, A., & Cannell, C. F. The effect of interviewer voice intonation on reporting, in Cannell, C. F., Oksenberg, L., and Converse, J. M. (Eds.), *Experiments in Interviewing Techniques: Field Experiments in Health Reporting, 1971–1977.* U.S. Department of Health, Education, and Welfare, Health Resources Administration, National Center for Health Services Research, DHEW Publication No. HRA 78-3204, 1977, pp. 201–204.

Barnard, K. E., & Eyres, S. J. (Eds.), *Child Health Assessment Part 2: The First Year of Life,* U.S. Department of Health, Education, and Welfare, Health Resources Administration, Division of Nursing, DHEW Publication No. HRA 79-25, 1979.

Batey, M. V. Acquiescent response set: A source of measurement error. *Western Journal of Nursing Research,* Summer, 1979, *1,* pp. 247–249.

Bloch, D. *Attitudes and Practices of Mothers in the Sex Education of Their Daughters.* Unpublished doctoral dissertation, University of California, Berkeley, 1970.

Buros, O. K. *The Eighth Mental Measurements Yearbook.* New Jersey: The Gryphon Press, 1978.

Byerly, E. The nurse-researcher as participant observer in a nursing setting, in Brink, P. (Ed.), *Transcultural Nursing: A Book of Readings.* Englewood Cliffs, New Jersey: Prentice-Hall, 1976, pp. 143–162.

Cannell, C. F., & Kahn, R. L. Interviewing, in Lindzey, G., & Aronson, E. (Eds.), *Handbook of Social Psychology,* 2nd edition, Vol. II. Reading, Massachusetts: Addison-Wesley, 1968, pp. 526–595.

Comrey, A. L., Becker, T. E., & Glaser, E. M. *A Sourcebook for Mental Health Measures.* Los Angeles: Human Interaction Research Institute, 1973.

Cromwell, L. & Arditt, M. *Medical Instrumentation for Health Care.* Englewood Cliffs, New Jersey: Prentice-Hall, 1976.

Dubowitz, L. M. S., Dubowitz, V., & Goldberg, C. Clinical assessment of gestational age in the newborn infant, *Journal of Pediatrics,* July, 1970, *77,* No. 1, pp. 2–10.

Edwards, A. L. *Techniques of Attitude Scale Construction.* New York: Appleton-Century-Crofts, 1957.

Geddes, L. A., & Baker, L. E. *Principles of Applied Biomedical Instrumentation.* New York: John Wiley & Sons, 1968.

Goldman, B. H. *Directory of Unpublished Experimental Mental Health Measures.* New York: Behavioral Publications, 1974.

Hollingshead, A. B. *Two Factor Index of Social Position.* New Haven, Connecticut: Privately Published. 1957.

Holsti, O. R. Content Analysis, in Lindzey, G. & Aronson, E. (Eds.), *Handbook of Social Psychology,* 2nd edition, Vol. II. Reading, Massachusetts: Addison-Wesley, 1968, pp. 596–692.

Hutt, S. J. & Hutt, C. *Direct Observation and Measurement of Behavior.* Springfield, Illinois: Charles C Thomas, 1970.

Jenkins, C. D. The semantic differential for health: A technique for measuring beliefs about diseases. *Public Health Reports,* June 1966, *81,* pp. 549–558.

Johnson, L., & Lubin, A. On planning psychophysiological experiments, in Greenfield, N. S., & Sternbach, R. A. (Eds.), *Handbook of Psychophysiology.* New York: Holt, Rinehart and Winston, 1972, pp. 125–158.

Johnson, O. G., & Bommarito, J. W. *Tests and Measurements in Child Development: A Handbook.* San Francisco: Jossey-Bass, 1971.

Kerlinger, F. N. *Foundations of Behavioral Research,* 2nd edition. New York: Holt, Rinehart and Winston, 1973.

Loustau, A., Lentz, M., Lee, K., McKenna, M., Hirako, S., Walker, W. F., & Wyman, J. The development of reliability of a clinical evaluation tool using student behavior recorded on videotape. *Journal of Nursing Education,* in press.

Meadow, L. & Gass, G. Z. Problems of the novice interviewer. *The American Journal of Nursing,* February, 1963, *63,* pp. 97–99.

Oppenheim, A. N. *Questionnaire Design and Attitude Measurement.* New York: Basic Books, 1966.

Palmer, I. S. The development of a measuring device: Measuring patients' perceptions toward impending surgery. *Nursing Research,* 1965, *14,* pp. 100–105.

Pascall, G. T., & Jenkins, W. O. *Systematic Observation of Gross Human Behavior.* New York: Grune & Stratton, 1961.

Robinson, J. P., Athansiou, R., Head, K. B. *Measures of Occupational Attitudes and Occupational Characteristics.* Ann Arbor: Survey Research Center, Institute of Social Research, 1969.

Robinson, J. P., Rusk, J. G., & Head, K. B. *Measures of Political Attitudes.* Ann Arbor: Survey Research Center, Institute of Social Research, 1968.

Robinson, J. P., & Shaver, P. R. *Measures of Social Psychological Attitude.* Ann Arbor: Survey Research Center, Institute of Social Research, 1973.

Sackett, G. P. (Ed.). *Observing Behavior, Vol. II: Data Collection and Methods.* NICHD Mental Research Centers Series. Baltimore: University Park Press, 1978.

Selltiz, C., Wrightsman, L. S., & Cook, S. W. *Research Methods in Social Relations,* 3rd edition. New York: Holt, Rinehart and Winston, 1976.

Smith, H. W. *Strategies of Social Research.* New Jersey: Prentice-Hall, 1975, pp. 60–61.

Snider, J. G., & Osgood, C. E. (Eds.). *Semantic Differential Technique.* Chicago: Aldine Publishing Company, 1969.

Strauss, M. A. *Family Measurement Techniques.* Minneapolis: University of Minnesota Press, 1969.

Ward, M. J., & Fetler, M. E. *Instruments for Use in Nursing Education Research.* Boulder, Colorado: Western Interstate Commission for Higher Education, 1979.

Ward, M. J., & Lindeman, C. A. *Instruments for Measuring Nursing Practice and Other Health Care Variables,* Vols. I and II. U.S. Department of Health, Education, and Welfare, Health Resources Administration, Bureau of Health Manpower, Division of Nursing, DHEW Publication No. HRA 78-54, 1978.

Weick, K. E. Systematic observation methods, in Lindzey, G., & Aronson, E. (Eds.), *Handbook of Social Psychology*, 2nd edition, Vol. II. Reading, Massachusetts: Addison-Wesley, 1968.

Williams, H. A. *Perceived Needs and Support Systems of Single Parents with Children Diagnosed with a Life-Threatening Illness.* Unpublished Master's thesis, University of Washington, Seattle 1979.

11 Questionnaire Development

Chapter 10 presented several methods for collecting data for a study. An additional important method for collecting data is the survey questionnaire. Survey questionnaires are frequently used in nursing research although their construction is difficult. Because a well-constructed questionnaire adds a great deal of strength to any study, understanding of questionnaire preparation is essential. This chapter presents an overview of the types of questionnaires that are relevant to nursing research and the interests of the nursing profession. Particular attention is given to the construction of a structured questionnaire.

Webster's defines a questionnaire as "a set of questions for obtaining statistically useful or personal information from individuals." Questionnaires are often used to collect facts, opinions, or beliefs of respondents (Selltiz, Wrightsman, and Cook, 1976). They are frequently called the test instruments. The form of a questionnaire may vary. It can be structured, unstructured, or a combination of both. In every case, it is necessary that informed consent be obtained from each respondent in advance.

TYPES OF QUESTIONNAIRES

Structured Questionnaires

Structured questionnaires are systematically organized to achieve a set of objectives. They are systems of wholes rather than aggregates of separate parts. That is, the questionnaire is constructed with an overall purpose in mind. The questions should flow directly from that purpose and follow each other in logical sequence. There is provided a choice of responses from which the subject makes a selection. For example, suppose a study purpose is to "determine the dietary knowledge of obese patients in a weight-loss program." The subjects may be asked,

"Which whole piece of fresh fruit has the highest number of calories?" The patients are given the following alternatives: apple, banana, orange, peach, plum. The correct answer is banana. All questions in this type of questionnaire would relate to the study purpose, and the answers would permit the investigator to draw conclusions about the dietary knowledge of the patients. If a large number of patients fail to identify the banana as having the highest number of calories, the director would rightly conclude that the weight-loss program needed revision. It may be important to present more information about the place of fruit in a weight-loss plan.

Another example of this type of questionnaire can be found in the examinations that many students must take in order to pass a course. These examinations often are a multiple choice type where the student is asked to select the one correct answer to a specific question. After careful attention to the construction of the test and a review of the student responses, the professor is able to draw conclusions about the weakness and strength of the material presented and what the students know or have learned. Clearly, the purpose of this type of questionnaire would be to determine the level of knowledge of a group of students about the material presented in a specific course. Course work revisions would be based on student performance in the examinations.

Unstructured Questionnaires

Unstructured questionnaires contain open-ended questions to which subjects are asked to write down responses in their own words. Subjects are not provided a list of alternative responses from which to choose a response. For example, suppose the researcher is interested in mothers' opinions about the nursing care that their hospitalized children receive. The researcher may distribute to the mothers a list of questions such as "Please explain how the nurse spends her time with your child." Several blank lines are left under the question so that the mothers may write down their own answers on the questionnaire. The researcher then analyzes the content of these responses on all the questionnaires in an effort to make some summary statements. The results are likely to be similar to opinion polls with a variety of answers. In this case it is difficult to make statistically valid conclusions.

Special Concerns in Developing Structured Questionnaires

Particular attention must be given to certain aspects in the development of structured questionnaires. To ensure that the questionnaires are understandable to the subjects and elicit the subjects' true responses, careful attention should be paid to the following aspects: 1) the language to be used in the questionnaire; 2) neutral wording; 3) the respondents' perception of the meaning of each question; and 4) memory and recall of the respondents. One or more illustrations of each of these considerations are presented in the following sections.

Language of the Questionnaire or Instrument

The language used in the instrument must be appropriate for the subjects and usually should be in their native language and idiom. If they are Spanish-speaking, Spanish would be the language. The subjects must be able to understand the meaning not only of the words but also of the intention of the question. A question that includes difficult words risks being misunderstood by the subjects, and the researcher may not get a valid response. (Selltiz, et al., 1976). For instance, suppose the researcher wanting to determine the personal goals of unmarried female nurses, asked the question "Identify the one item that best incorporates your personal goals: a) higher educational degree; b) financial success; c) job security; d) job advancement; e) marriage." The respondent may not be able to choose among these alternatives because they overlap too much (marriage and financial success) or because they are equally important. Further, the respondent may have other important personal goals, such as maintaining good health. A better list of alternatives would be one that eliminates overlap so that the respondent could more easily select one answer from the list or one that includes an "other———" category, in which the respondent supplies his or her own answer.

Neutral Wording

To the extent possible, words, phrases, and sentences in the questionnaire should be free of bias. Certain value words, such as hate, love, disgusting, admire, and abhor, can imply the type of response that is expected or desired. Asking a "yes-no" question such as "Did you hate the nursing care that you received in the hospital?" probably will not be reliably answered by the patient and probably cannot be answered in unequivocal terms. The patient might also be concerned for possible reprisals. A better and neutral question would be "Do you believe you received adequate nursing care? If no, specify deficiency———." This question can be answered by yes or no, and the follow-up probe provides an example and explanation. All leading questions that imply or invite certain answers are to be avoided.

Stereotyped Responses and Opinions

Many people have acquired rigid and stereotyped opinions from experience, television, radio, journals, or the comments of others. To minimize responses based on these stereotyped opinions, questions must be phrased to avoid current jargon and conventional wisdom. By sharpening the contrast among alternative responses, subjects can be encouraged to think and to give their own truthful responses. The possibility of spurious or untruthful responses must always be kept in mind and efforts made to minimize them.

Memory and Recall

Because peoples' memories are both fallible and limited, questions should deal with fairly recent events. Experience has shown that events that occurred even two weeks or longer before the time of a questionnaire are not recalled with full accuracy. The longer the recall interval, the less accurate is the memory.

ADMINISTERING A QUESTIONNAIRE

Structured questionnaires may be self-administered. They may be distributed at the bedside of hospitalized patients, handed to patients in an out-patient department clinic, or given to students for a course evaluation. They also may be mailed to the subjects. In these cases, the respondent completes the questionnaire without the aid of another person. Pilot studies can be completed to determine whether differences occur as a result of various methods of questionnaire administration.

Questionnaires may also be self-administered in the presence of an interviewer or research assistant. The respondent answers the questions, but the interviewer is available to answer any queries for clarification. However, self-administered questionnaires that are completed with the aid of an interviewer involve special considerations. First, the interviewer should be trained in appropriate methods. Specifically the interviewer should know what questions to ask and how to answer questions (Payne, 1951). Because the training of interviewers may be time-consuming and delay the completion of the study, discretion should be used. Interviewers should not be used with self-administered questionnaires without good reason.

A second and more serious problem is that the interviewer may introduce bias into a subject's responses (Hulka, Zyzanski, and Cassel, 1970; Brink and Wood, 1978). Hoping to please the interviewer, the subject may respond in socially acceptable ways and may avoid expressing negative attitudes. The respondent may attempt to impress the interviewer with the level of satisfaction by giving only favorable responses. The reverse may also be true. In either situation the interviewer cannot be certain about the validity of the patient responses. If the researcher wants to collect data from a hospitalized patient, the interviewer would be specially instructed in the methods of approaching and questioning hospitalized patients. The interviewer would be asked to carry the instrument to the bedside of the patient and wait while it is completed. The interviewer would be asked to pay close attention to the amount of probing and clarifying that accompanies the data collection process. Further, the interviewer would be instructed to report any untoward responses to the researcher so that interviewer-patient problems could be identified and resolved. The greatest advantage in the use of interviewers is the likelihood of obtaining a high response rate.

Questionnaires can be administered in several ways or combinations of ways. The questions can be printed on a form and the subject asked to write the answers. An interviewer may ask the prescribed questions orally and write down the oral answers of the subjects. The questions may be asked orally and the alternative answers may be printed on a card presented to the subject who will then answer orally. Details for administering questionnaires may be found in any social research methods text (such as Selltiz, et al., 1976).

Informed Consent

When people are asked to participate in research, they must be given the opportunity to consent or to refuse to become a subject. Whether or not these people are under the care of institutions such as hospitals, nursing homes, or schools, they must be told that any research to be conducted in or through that agency has been reviewed and approved by an appropriate committee concerned with research ethics. Emotional and physical well-being of the subjects are the prime concerns of these committees.

Only after agency approval has been gained is the researcher free to begin data collection. However, in order to proceed ethically, the researcher must ask each subject to consent to participate in the study. This consent may be obtained through a verbal agreement or preferably with the subject's signature. In either case, the subject must be informed of the study purpose, any risks involved, and the length of time required. The subject must be assured that privacy will be observed and that no subject will be specifically identified (see Chap. 2).

Rather than having the subject read a form that includes all of the above information, the interviewer may explain the study briefly, answer any questions, and then request the subject to sign a consent form. This form would include, for example, a statement such as "This study (title) has been explained to me and I agree to participate." The subject would be asked to sign name and date underneath such a statement. After explaining the study and obtaining the signature or verbal consent, the researcher may proceed with the study.

If the consent is verbal, the interviewer should record the fact on the questionnaire form with the date. Even though writing answers to questions or giving answers to questions orally implies consent, it is preferable to have the consent made explicit in writing.

Most subjects may have little or no interest in knowing about the research findings of a study. However, if the subjects are interested, the researcher is obligated to send them a report of the findings of the research in which they participated.

Response Rates

The response rates of subjects participating in studies are of major importance for a successful study. If the response rate is too low, no valid conclusion can be drawn. The rates tend to differ according to the methods used for data collection. The highest response rates can be expected when questionnaires are self-administered with the aid of an interviewer. It seems clear that subjects will respond more readily and completely when interviewers are present. Not only are interviewers able to gain consent from subjects and collect the questionnaires immediately upon completion, but also prospective subjects who are unwilling to participate in the study make their refusal known immediately. Experience has shown that response rates tend to be good using this method.

Mailed questionnaires, on the other hand, usually yield lower response rates. These mailed packets should include, in addition to the questionnaire, a covering letter that explains the study and the questionnaire and gives a deadline date for the questionnaire's return. A pre-addressed stamped envelope should also be included for the subject to use to return the questionnaire. The response is left entirely to the subject, and the investigator should not expect a very high return rate. Thirty percent is a good first response to a mailed questionnaire.

When there are a large number of nonresponses with the use of mailed questionnaires, the researcher may encourage a higher response rate by sending a second mailing of the questionnaire, reminder letters, post cards, or phone calls. These efforts may serve to foster interest in the study and thus result in a return of the completed questionnaires. However, even these nudges may not yield an adequate return rate, which should be at least 75% or higher.

Usually, high response rates are achieved when data are collected through questionnaires administered by trained interviewers. With this method, a smaller sample size may be needed than for the mailed questionnaires, which require a larger sample size because of poorer response rates. However, the mailed questionnaires are relatively fast to distribute and therefore are usually less expensive to administer. All of these factors must be considered when planning the method of data collection for a study.

CONSTRUCTING A QUESTIONNAIRE TO MEASURE PATIENT PERCEPTIONS

This section presents a study of the process used for the development of a structured questionnaire to measure perceptions (rather than attitudes, beliefs, knowledge) of people about their needs (Williamson, 1978). The purposes of the study were to:

1. Describe patients' definitions of their needs during hospitalization (a) soon after admission and (b) at the time of discharge.
2. Investigate the extent to which patients' definitions of their needs were similar to nurses' definitions of the patients' needs.
3. Examine the congruence of nurse and patient perceptions of patient needs and the congruence between patient satisfactions with nursing care and nurse satisfactions with the care given.

The development of a questionnaire for the second study purpose is the focus of this section. The study was carefully planned in its design, definitions, hypotheses, analysis, and so forth, before the questionnaire development began.

The purposes of the questionnaire in this example were to collect background information on the patients and the nurses participating in the study and the perceptions of both groups about the patients' needs. In order to satisfy these purposes the questionnaire was divided into two parts. Part I was a personal data section used to collect information on the characteristics of the patient and nurse respondents. Part II, the major aspect of the questionnaire, was designed to obtain information on the perceptions of the patients and of the nurses regarding patients' needs. This process of questionnaire development is described in the next two sections.

Part I: Personal Data Items

The first step was to prepare a personal data form. This form was used to collect background information about the study participants. The forms were required to be brief, that is, relatively easy to complete, and the content *directly* related to the study purpose. In this study the background information for the *patients* included

1. Birthdate, sex, marital status, ethnic background
2. Admission date
3. Educational level
4. Perceived health problems
5. Previous hospitalizations
6. Distance from home to the hospital (in miles)
7. Admission diagnosis

The personal data form for the *nurses* included

1. Birthdate, sex, marital status
2. Type of nursing education (associate degree, diploma, or baccalaureate degree)
3. Years of experience as a staff nurse
4. Years of experience in that clinical setting
5. Usual shift assignment

This form was pretested on patients and nurses to make certain that it was clearly written. If it were not satisfactory, it would have had to be edited and pretested again, and the process continued until the investigator was confident that the form was clear and adequate.

Analysis of the personal data would provide information about how similar or dissimilar the patients were and how similar or dissimilar the nurses were. Unless each group was reasonably homogeneous, drawing valid conclusions would have been difficult. Variations among patients and among nurses would help to explain or understand variations in their perceptions of needs and wants.

Part II: Development of Patient Needs and Wants Items

An initial list of patient needs was developed through a literature review and interviews with clinical specialists in nursing. Ten patient needs were identified by this process, as follows:

1. To be assured that the physician's orders will be carefully and expertly carried out
2. To be provided with physical assistance until able to assume responsibility for self-care in part or in full
3. To know that meals will be served promptly

4. To be provided with a clean and restful environment
5. To know that the nurse will respond quickly to pain or discomforts
6. To be assured of consistent and continuous nursing care
7. To receive individualized personal care
8. To be surrounded by warm and friendly nurses
9. To have time for talking with the nurses
10. To be allowed to make decisions about self-care when it is appropriate

Those ten items then were reviewed by registered nurses, discharged patients, and lay people for their understanding of the meaning of the items. Two classifications of needs emerged: identifiable physical needs and identifiable emotional needs. Revisions of the needs lists, based on the comments and interpretations, are listed below under the two classifications.

A. Physical needs
   1. Assistance with self-care until able to do it alone
   2. Clean environment
   3. Prompt relief from discomfort
   4. Physician's orders carried out accurately
   5. Appropriate meals at appropriate times
   6. Adequate rest during hospitalization

B. Emotional needs
   1. Having pleasant people providing the care
   2. Having personalized care
   3. Having family members or close friends informed of the treatment plan
   4. Receiving explanations about hospital routines
   5. Receiving explanations about hospital policies
   6. Getting answers to questions about the illness and treatment
   7. Having an opportunity to talk about problems to someone who listens
   8. Having knowledgeable people providing care

To develop more precise items, these 14 general needs were expanded into 36 specific needs: 15 physical needs and 21 emotional needs. The items then were pretested on at least five patients per item, as recommended by Nunnally (1967). These patients were chosen to be as representative of the study group as possible. Each patient was asked to rate each of the 36 needs as to its importance, using a Likert type scale: 1 = always important; 2 = almost always important; 3 = sometimes important; 4 = seldom important; 5 = not important. For a full discussion of the Likert scale and others, such as the Thurston and Semantic Differential Scales, see Nachmias (1976) and Selltiz, et al. (1976).

When clear and satisfactorily stated, these 36 needs (items) were used to create the questionnaire item list, which then was administered to a pretest group and as soon thereafter as possible to a group similar to the study group. Data were collected from both groups within a brief period of time by the same person. This helped to eliminate possible problems related to the validity of the questionnaire. An item analysis then was conducted by comparing the responses of the two groups. From this comparison it was possible to determine which of the items for each concept were the most reliable, that is, those items which showed the most consistent responses.

Item Analysis

Responses to the 36 items were analyzed for item reliability using Pearson's Product-Moment Correlation (r) (Blalock, 1972). Those items having the lowest mean r values were eliminated because the responses did not correlate well with each other and therefore the items were not considered reliable. Cronback's alpha (α) was also calculated to measure the internal consistency of the remaining 11 physical needs (α = .77) and 17 emotional needs (α = .89). Statistically, these scores indicated the degree of agreement of the items within each of the two classifications. Correlation values show more reliability as they approach 1.0 (Bohrnstedt, 1970).

As a final step in developing a list of needs that were considered reliable, item-to-total correlations were calculated for

1. Each physical item to total physical needs
2. Each emotional item to total emotional needs
3. Each physical item to total emotional needs
4. Each emotional item to total physical needs

The items were then inspected again using Cronback's alpha. Those physical items that correlated highly with the total emotional needs in (3) and those emotional items that correlated highly with total physical needs in (4) were eliminated because they did not reflect the appropriate concept. Also, those items in (1) and (2) above with low correlations were eliminated.

Physical

1. Assistance in self-care until able to do it alone
2. Receive correct diet
3. Have a comfortable bed
4. Receive food at the usual meal times

Emotional

5. Receive help from people who seem happy to care for the patient
6. Receive care from people who know patient's name
7. Receive information about patient's treatments and procedures
8. Have an opportunity to share worries with someone who listens

TESTING FOR VALIDITY AND RELIABILITY

In developing a reliable and valid patient need scale, it is important to remember that it can be strengthened if the sample, time, place, and researchers (interviewers) are similar for the pretest and for the study groups (Selltiz, et al., 1976). If this is not done, the researcher may discover important statistical differences between the pretest respondents and the study group respondents, as a result of researcher differences. Differences in the responses also may be explained if the researcher compares demographic characteristics of the two groups. The item list and reliability should be pretested on as many as possible of the types of subjects who would be included in the eventual study group. Pretesting subjects in the same setting in which the eventual study would be conducted or in a setting that is similar would help to minimize differences. Further, there should be a relatively short period of time, two to four weeks, between the pretest and time of actual data collection for the study.

Although there are many possible problems, it is clear that the most serious problems relate to concept measurement and study design. Much time must be devoted to sharpening the concept under study and preparing the test instrument. The investigator must make certain that the concepts are distinct and do not overlap. In the example of the patients' needs study, subjects may not have differentiated between physical and emotional needs when they responded. For instance, a need such as to "receive the correct diet" might be interpreted as an emotional rather than a physical need. This becomes more understandable when considering a patient with ulcerative colitis, who would be concerned about receiving the correct diet from both the physical and emotional need aspects. The researcher might have difficulty differentiating between the two needs. This problem could be avoided if the researcher studied only one group of patients with the same diagnosis or the same illness.

CONDUCTING THE STUDY

When the final list of reliable items for perceived patient needs has been developed, the format of the questionnaire would be prepared. The personal data section should precede the patient needs section. In this way the subject is asked to respond first to questions that are familiar and easy to answer. Part II of the questionnaire usually requires more thought and more of the respondent's time.

Then, the individuals in the study group—patients and nurses—would be asked to complete the questionnaire. Each respondent would be asked to rate each item according to how important it is, or is thought to be, to the patient. The Likert scale would be used again as in the pretest. An interviewer assisting in the collection of these data is helpful to the respondent as well as to the investigator. The questionnaire should be administered to study subjects at the times that are relevant to the study purpose. In this example, it was administered to patients and nurses at the times of the patients' admission and again at the time of the patients' discharge from the hospital. The time of questionnaire administration was related to subjects' perceptions and how they might change during the course of hospitalization.

By statistical analysis of the responses, it is possible to make valid interpretations of the degree of congruence between patients' and nurses' perceptions of need and whether patients' perceptions change between the time of admission and the time shortly before discharge.

It is clear that certain questions considered in the construction of any reliable and valid patient need scale would be useful for many types of hospitalized patients. The concepts of physical and emotional needs, however, require elaboration and refinement. Items selected to be included in a reliable measuring instrument would need to be not only specific to each concept but also sensitive to different types of patients. Additionally, thoughtful consideration would have to be given to the following questions: (1) What is the objective with respect to generalizability of the findings? (2) What is the most appropriate method for selecting the sample of patients? (3) What demographic characteristics of the patients are important to identify? A fuller identification of the needs of the different patients who are admitted to hospitals with many different health disorders is suggested as a starting point.

SUMMARY

This chapter has presented a discussion of two types of questionnaires. These types are unstructured and structured. Attention was given to two methods of questionnaire administration: self-administered and administered by interviewers. Problems and some solutions for each of these methods were identified. Special focus in this chapter was given to the process of developing a structured questionnaire, and an example was provided.

BIBLIOGRAPHY

Blalock, H. M. *Social Statistics.* New York: McGraw-Hill, 1972.

Bohrnstedt, G. W. Reliability and validity assessment in attitude measurement in Summers, G. F. (Ed.), *Attitude Measurement.* Chicago: Rand-McNally, 1970.

Brink, P. J., & Wood, M. J. *Basic Steps in Planning Nursing Research.* Scituate, Massachusetts: Duxbury Press, 1978.

Hulka, B. S., Zyzanski, S. J., Cassel, J. C., & Thompson, C. J. Scale for the measurement of attitudes toward physicians and primary medical care. *Medical Care* September/October, 1970, *8,* No. 5, pp. 429–436.

Nachmias, D., Nachmias, C. *Research Methods in the Social Sciences.* New York: St. Martin's Press, 1976.

Nunnally, J. C. *Psychometric Theory.* New York: McGraw-Hill, 1967.

Payne, S. L. *The Art of Asking Questions.* Princeton, New Jersey: Princeton University Press, 1951.

Selltiz, C., Wrightsman, L. S., & Cook, S. W. *Research Methods in Social Relations,* 3rd edition. New York: Holt, Rinehart and Winston, 1976.

Williamson, Y. M. Methodologic dilemmas in tapping the concept of patient needs. *Nursing Research,* May/June, 1978, *27,* No. 3, pp. 172–177.

Part 4

ANALYSIS AND REPORTING OF COLLECTED RESEARCH DATA

Part 4 describes the culmination of the nurse's research efforts by explaining methods of describing, analyzing, and reporting information about the collected data. The first aspect of this process is presented in Chapter 12, in which methods for the statistical description of the attributes of samples are discussed. Upon completion of this chapter, the student will have gained knowledge about measures of central tendency and dispersion, distribution curves, and frequency distributions. The importance of this information for describing data will be apparent. Chapter 13 introduces in the first section some of the parametric statistical techniques that may be used for samples. These methods will allow the student to make inferences about the population from which the sample was drawn. The second section of Chapter 13 presents selected nonparametric statistical procedures that may be used for samples with restricted assumptions about their origins. Chapters 12 and 13 form the basis for Chapter 14, which outlines the content that is necessary to include in a presentation of the findings of a study. The chapter describes ways in which the data can be organized for presentation, as well as questions that should be addressed so that the findings are shown in a context that allows for assessment of their value. Research contributions to nursing knowledge are the ultimate goals.

Finally, Chapter 15 describes a method for critiquing research articles and reporting a study in article form for publication in journals. This chapter provides an opportunity for the student to integrate the information presented in Part 4 as well as the information introduced in previous chapters. Overall, Part 4 contains the information the student needs to reach the goal of conducting research that is based not only on knowledge but also on scholarly efforts.

12
Descriptive Statistics

Statistics is the science of assembling, classifying, tabulating, and analyzing numerical data related to samples. Chapter 10 presented methods of assembling and classifying data. This chapter discusses methods for statistically describing data once they have been collected, assembled, and classified. Measures of central tendency, measures of dispersion, and distribution curves are the primary focus of the chapter. These values provide a meaningful basis for describing collected information by placing the sample data into a framework that is easily understood by other people.

Studies that rely on descriptive statistics are those that portray details about the sample, setting, variables, and so on, so that the findings can be used to help explain similarities or differences among those factors. Further, based on the observed data, these methods allow us to make inferences or predictions about the general situation under study.

MEASURES OF CENTRAL TENDENCY

Central tendency, one of the most important concepts in statistics, may be defined as the distinctive quality of a distribution to aggregate or concentrate around particular numerical values. In other words, the values automatically will form some type of distribution. This distribution can then be described by specific measures, including the mean, mode, and median of an array of values. These measures are the most frequently used and most easily understood descriptive statistics.

Mean

The mean, ($\bar{X}$) or more accurately the arithmetic mean, is the average of a group of values. It is the most stable of the measures and is used in everyday life. For example, measuring average daily temperatures and average miles per gallon of gasoline are familiar expressions of weather conditions or automobile efficiency. In research the mean serves a similar function by telling us, for example, the average age of a group of respondents, average length of hospital stay, average number of times a particular item was selected as most important on a questionnaire, or whatever is relevant to the research question. The investigator gains a sense of those average values relevant to the subjects regarding their ages, responses, length of hospitalization, and so on. Thus, he or she is in a position to compare the findings with those of other groups who may have been asked to respond to similar research questions.

Calculating the mean of a group of observations tells us the center of gravity of those values. It is a value so determined that the sum of the positive deviations from it is equal to the sum of the negative deviations. This process is discussed fully in the section on measures of dispersion. The usual method of calculating the mean is illustrated in the following example. Suppose we have a group of 8(N) test scores in which some of the scores are earned by more than one student (f). The highest possible score is 25. The notations are: X = test score, f = frequency of the score, or the number of students who earn it, fx = the score times the frequency, N = the number of students, $\overline{X}$ = mean, Σ = sum.

X	f	fx
22	4	88
20	3	60
15	1	15
	$N = 8$	$\Sigma fx = 163$

The following formula is used to calculate the mean ($\overline{X}$) of these scores:

$$\overline{X} = \frac{\Sigma fx}{N} = \frac{163}{8} = 20.38$$

Hence, we can say that the average score on this test was 20.38. Students are able to evaluate their performance on the test in relation to the class average.

The average test score in this example is usually calculated as the arithmetic average (mean). Without care in reporting, however, some people may interpret the average score as the most frequent occurrence of the score (mode) or the middle score (median) of the test. The mode and median give different information; they indicate the position of certain scores in the full array of scores.

Mode

The mode in a distribution of values or scores is the score that occurs most often. It *need not* fall in the center of a distribution of values. In the example discussed above, the mode is 22. More students earned that score than any other score. The mode of this test is an important value for the instructor to know. It may indicate that the test was too easy and in need of revision. The same data inspection and revision may apply in health care, nursing care, and so on. The modal length of time of patients under hospital care may indicate a need to evaluate the type of care given. Perhaps nursing care could be more efficient.

Median

The median (M) is the point in the distribution above or below which 50% of the frequencies lie. In order for the median to be calculated, the values must be arranged in ascending or descending order. In the example of the test, scores are arranged in descending order. The formula for calculating the median of the scores is

$$\text{Median} = \frac{\text{Total Count } (N = 8)\ \downarrow}{\uparrow\ 2 \rightarrow \qquad \text{grows to}}$$

Whole numbers grow halfway to the next integer. Hence $8/2 = 4$ grows to 4.5. This number tells us that the median of the distribution is the 4.5th score in the array.

After arranging the numbers in descending or ascending order, we find that the median lies between the scores of 22 and 20 in the distribution:

22
22
22
22
$\leftarrow M = 21$
20
20
20
15
$\Sigma = 163$

We would average these two scores $(22 + 20)/2$ and determine that the median of this test is at the score of 21.0.

This example illustrates the method for calculating the median when we have an even number (8) of integers in the array. However, this is not always the case. If we had had an odd number of integers in the array, for example 7, and the array did not contain the score of 15, we would have had

$$M = \frac{7}{2} = 3.5 \text{ grows to 4 and therefore } M = 22.$$

Nonintegers grow to the next larger integer. Thus 3.5 grows to 4 and the median is the fourth score in the array. Counting four scores, we find that the median is 22.

Plotting the mean, median, and mode of these test scores in a frequency polygon permits the inspection of the varying positions of the mean, mode, and median, as seen in Figure 12-1. These values clearly do not resemble a normal curve because the large number of high scores (mode = 22) skew the distribution in a negative direction (left) in relation to the mean. The polygon shows the different positions of the three measures of central tendency for these eight scores. This example is presented purposely using a small N so that we can gain an understanding of the relationship of these measures to each other in the simplest framework. A larger sample size may or may not show that the relationships would be identical. However, if the distribution were normal, they would be identical (see the "Normal Curves" section of this chapter).

MEASURES OF DISPERSION

In the preceding section we presented measures of central tendency that allow us to describe data from that perspective. This section discusses the measures of dispersion that are used to describe how data depart from their centrality. Standard deviation, variance and range are those measures.

Standard Deviation

The standard deviation (SD) is an estimate of how much all the individual values deviate from the group mean. It is a summary measure of the differences of each value from the mean. When these differences are summed, the negative values and the positive values balance each other, and their sum is zero.

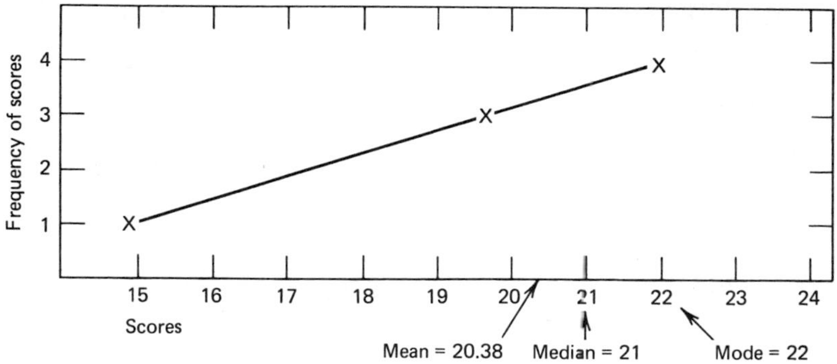

Figure 12-1. Illustration of mean, median and mode of nursing student test scores.

Two formulas may be used for calculating the standard deviation of a group of values. These are the definitional formula,

$$SD = \sqrt{\frac{\Sigma(X - \bar{X})^2}{N - 1}},$$

and the calculating formula, where x = the variance,

$$SD = \sqrt{\frac{\Sigma x^2}{N} - \bar{X}^2}.$$

Examples of calculating the standard deviation are presented, first using the definitional formula and then the calculating formula.

Suppose we are interested in determining the SD of the length of waiting time (in minutes) that eight patients experienced before they saw the physician. Table 12-1 illustrates the method using the definitional formula.

We determine that the SD = 7.74 minutes.

Table 12-2 illustrates the use of the calculating formula with these same values.

The difference in the standard deviation values in the two methods is due to the subtraction of 1 from N ($N - 1$) in the denominator of the definitional formula. This is an unbiased estimate of the standard deviation and is used when there are a small number of values. The calculating formula clearly is less laborious than the definitional for-

Table 12-1. Use of Definitional Formula for the Standard Deviation[a]

Waiting Time In Minutes X	f	$\bar{X}$	$X - \bar{X}$	$(X - \bar{X})^2$
38	1	26.13	11.87	141.02
35	1		8.87	78.77
30	1		3.87	15.01
25	1		−1.13	1.27
24	1		−2.13	4.52
22	1		−4.13	17.02
20	1		−6.13	37.52
15	1		−11.13	123.77
$\Sigma X = 209$	$N = 8$		0	$\Sigma(X - \bar{X})^2 = 418.9$

$\bar{X} = 209/8 = 26.13$

[a]Using the definitional formula, SD $= \sqrt{418.9/7} = \sqrt{59.84} = 7.74$

mula. This is especially true with the use of a calculator for a large number of values. Note that:

$$\Sigma X^2 - \bar{X}^2 = \Sigma(X - \bar{X})^2$$

In these examples a standard deviation of 7.22 minutes tells us that a patient in this group had to wait about seven minutes more or seven minutes less than the average waiting time experienced by the patients.

Suppose we had an N of 18 and frequencies of more than 1 for some of the waiting times. In that instance we would multiply the frequency (f) times the waiting time (X) and determine fx. Table 12-3 illustrates the process for calculating the standard deviation under these circumstances.

Note that the mean is larger and the standard deviation is smaller when we have increased the size of N. Plotting these values on a curve, we note that the distribution does not appear to be normal (see Fig. 12-2).

Variance

Another measure of dispersion, variance, is defined as the standard deviation squared. It indicates dispersion from the mean in both the positive and negative directions. Recall that the standard deviation gives the dispersion of values from the mean in one direction only. In the preceding example the standard deviation is 7.22; hence the variance would equal 52.13. If we were to draw an infinite number of samples from the same population, the mean of each sample would be an estimate of the population mean. All those sample means would not be identical; however, their pattern would constitute a normal distribution. Their standard deviation, from this distribution is called the standard error of the mean.

Range

Range is the difference between the highest and lowest values in an observation. In the example of waiting times the range would be 38 − 15 = 23 minutes. Note that this time is 3 minutes less than the mean. In our example using frequencies of more than 1, the range would still be 23 minutes. This range still approximates the mean of 26.22, but the reader does not gain an understanding of the role that large frequencies play in that distribution. The range gives limited information as a measure of dispersion.

DISTRIBUTION CURVES

The framework for statistics lies in the concept of frequency distribution curves. These curves, in essence, give a pictorial display of data that reveals their location with respect to each other and to the theoretical normal curve.

Table 12-2. Use of Calculating Formula for the Standard Deviation[a]

X	X^2
38	1444
35	1225
30	900
25	625
24	576
22	484
20	400
15	225

$\Sigma x^2 = 5879 =$ sum of squares

[a]Using the calculating formula:
$SD = \sqrt{(\Sigma x^2/N) - \overline{X}^2} = \sqrt{(5879/8) - 682.78} = \sqrt{734.88 - 682.78} = \sqrt{52.10} = 7.22$.

Table 12-3. Standard Deviation Calculation for Frequencies of More Than One

X	f	fx	X^2
38	1	38	1444
35	2	70	2450
30	3	90	2700
25	3	75	1875
24	5	120	2880
22	2	44	968
20	1	20	400
15	1	15	225

N = 18 $\Sigma fx = 472$ $\Sigma X^2 = 12{,}942$

$N = 18$
$\bar{X} = 472/18 = 26.22$
$\Sigma fx = 472$
$\Sigma X^2 = 222{,}784$
$\Sigma x^2 = 12{,}942 - 12{,}376.98 = 565.02$

$\Sigma X^2 = 12{,}942$
$(\Sigma X)^2/N = 12{,}376.89$

$$SD = \sqrt{565.02/18} = 13.39$$
$$SD = 5.60$$

Collected data are described as being either discrete or continuous. Discrete data are those variables that can take on only a limited number of values. These are values that result, for example, from a count of numbers such as the number of patients a nurse cares for on her eight-hour work shift or the number of children who fail to keep appointments for immunizations. Another common example is the toss of a coin, the outcome of which can be only heads or tails. In this case the outcomes are mutually exclusive. Only one outcome can occur with each toss of a coin. The probability of each outcome remains constant over repeated independent tosses.

Continuous data are data whose values may assume any number of places on a measurement tool. Examples would include people's heights, weights, ages. In these instances the values could assume a variety of positions on the measurement continuum. The use of decimal places with the integers makes this variation possible. Whether data are continuous or discrete, they can be analyzed by their appropriate sampling distributions.

Sampling distributions constitute the basis for estimating the outcome of statistical tests. The distributions have been derived from drawing many samples from the same population and calculating their means. The distributions then form a backdrop against which we can evaluate or expect a particular outcome in a large number of experiments. They give us the theoretical distribution of all possible values of an estimate. Most statistics have sampling distributions and usually these are found in the appendices of statistics textbooks. This text includes sampling distributions for the *Z* scores, *t*-test, chi-square, and Spearman's rank correlation coefficient (see Appendix).

Normal Curves

The normal curve, used for continuous data, is one of the most important frequency distributions in statistics. This distribution was first described by DeMoivre in 1733 (Snedecor and Cochran, 1972). About 150 years ago it was further developed by Gauss and is frequently called the Gaussian distribution (Duncan, Knapp, and Miller, 1977). Normal does not mean "usual" or "everyday" (Dixon and Massey, 1969). This text uses the term normal distribution because it is more commonly used in nursing literature.

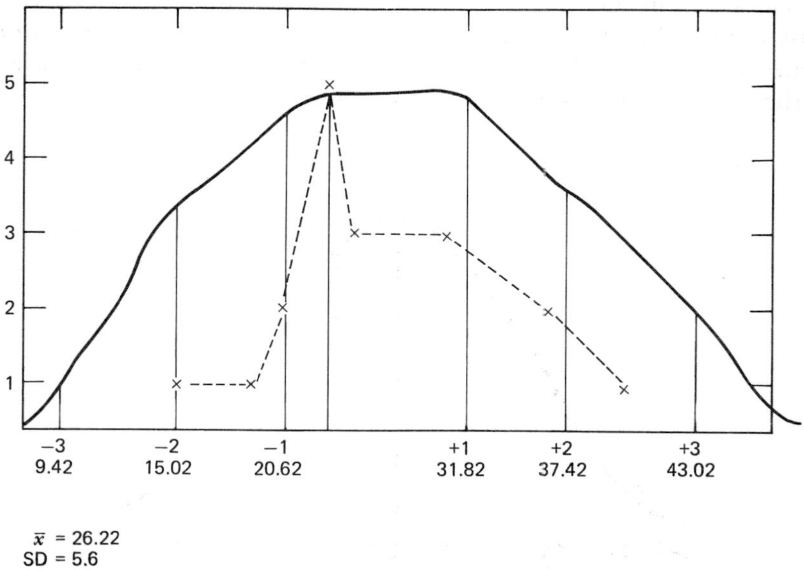

Figure 12-2. Frequency polygon of waiting times of 18 patients before physician visit.

When plotted, the frequencies of the normal distribution resemble a bell, often called the bell-shaped curve. It is symmetrical and unimodal and extends infinitely in both positive and negative directions with most of the values clustering in the center. The standard normal distribution has a mean of 0 and a standard deviation of 1, and its mean, mode, and median coincide (Fig. 12-3) (Blalock, 1972).

The area under the standard normal curve $N(0,1)$ may be inspected by the percent of values that lie between the standard deviation ordinates. That is

$$-1 \text{ to } +1 = 68.26\%$$

$$-1.96 \text{ to } +1.96 = 95.36\%$$

$$-2.58 \text{ to } +2.58 = 99.72\%$$

For ease of handling we round 1.96 to 2 and 2.58 to 3. Note that the area from −3 to +3 does not include 100% of the values, illustrating the theoretical concept of infinity in the tails in the curve.

Once data are plotted on a curve, we are able to ascertain their distribution in relation to the normal distribution. For example, if we determine that most of our values lie between −1 and +1 standard deviations from the mean, we would know that 68.26% of our values cluster about the center of gravity. We would then inspect our remaining values to determine their relative position to the mean. This application of the normal curve is used in many types of measurement.

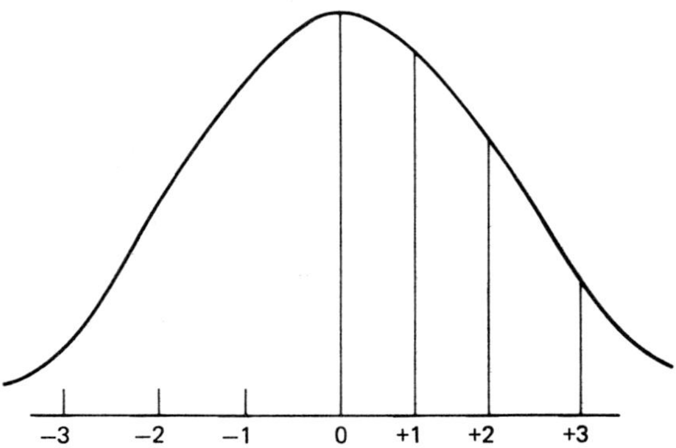

Figure 12-3. Normal curve: unimodal.

The normal curve occupies a central role in the techniques for performing statistical inferences. The key to its use is the standard score, Z. Standardized variables are based on the frequency distributions of sample means. Statistical theory shows that "the frequency distribution of $\overline{X}$ in repeat random samples of size n tends to become more normal as n increases" (Snedecor and Cochran, 1972, p. 51). This is the *Central Limit theorem,* and it underlies the theoretical normal distribution. As can be seen in Figure 12-3, approximation to normal improves as the sample size increases. A Z score is the position of a value in relation to the mean of many sample means. If repeated random samples of size n are drawn from any population (normal or not) that has a mean μ and a standard deviation σ, the frequency distribution of the sample mean $\bar{x}$ in repeated samples has a mean μ and a standard deviation σ/n and is normally distributed as n grows toward infinity. (See Appendix, Table A.) This fact tells us that with random sampling, the sample mean is an unbiased estimator of the population mean μ. The $\bar{x}$ is that point above and below which 50% of the data lie. The standard deviations are ± 1.96 and ± 2.58 (rounded to 2 and 3 standard deviations) from the mean. If we square the standard deviation (σ), we have the area under the curve from the mean in both directions. This is called the variance (σ^2). Figure 12-3 illustrates the relative total area under the curve of each population size. If the three populations had been the same size and had equal means but different standard deviations, the curve with the smaller deviations would be more peaked at the mean than the other two (Fig. 12-4). This observation becomes clear when we consider the concept of the distribution of normal curves.

In order to use the normal curve for data analysis, we standardize the data using the Z score. The standard Z score tells the number of standard deviations that an observation lies away from the population mean. To determine this distance, the raw data are converted to the Z score using the following formula:

$$Z = \frac{X - \overline{X}}{s}$$

where X is each raw data score, $\overline{X}$ is the sample mean, and s is the sample standard deviation.

To illustrate the process, suppose we have a group of 200 test results, with a mean test score of 50 and a standard deviation of 10. Converting each test score to a Z score is one way of determining whether the

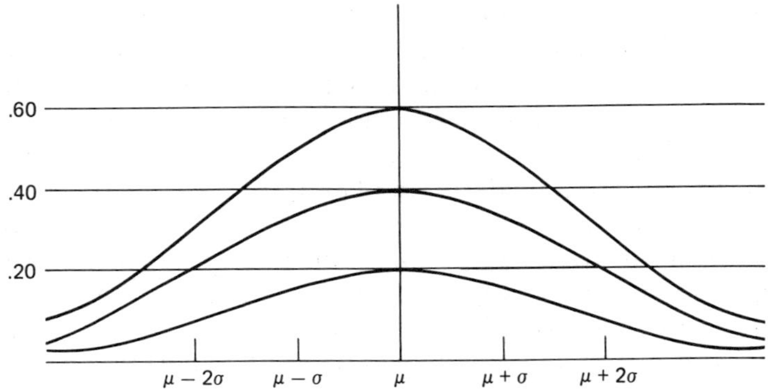

Figure 12-4. Distribution of population curves with equal means standard deviations and unequal sizes.

scores approximate normality. Using the Z score to convert the observed test score of 72, as an example, we find

$$Z = \frac{72 - 50}{10} = \frac{22}{10} = 2.2$$

Determining that we have a Z score of 2.2, we refer to the cumulative normal distribution table. This gives the percent of the population lying equal to or within the score. The Z value for this score lies .4865 to the right of the mean. When data are distributed normally, we say that 95% of the observations (scores) fall within 1.96 of the mean and 99% fall within 2.58 of the mean.

Nonnormal Curves

Many statistics have large numbers and, as stated, their sampling distributions are normal. However, this is not always the case. Samples may have been drawn from populations that do not have a normal distribution. In these instances the distributions may have two or more major clusters of values. Thus, they may be bimodal (Fig. 12-5) or trimodal (Fig. 12-6). There are rarely more than two or three modes in a distribution.

A further characteristic of a curve is the dispersion of frequency values around their center of gravity. As indicated in Figure 12-3, both tails of the curve are approximately the same size. A similar number of

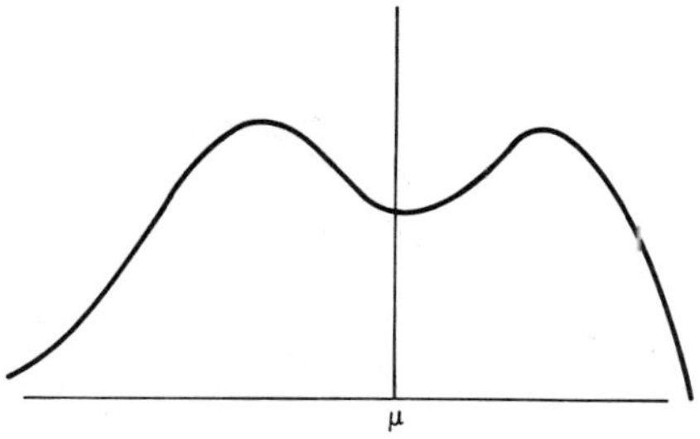

Figure 12-5. Bimodal curve.

values fall into each tail. However, this need not necessarily be the case. The values may group into one or the other of the two tails so that the distribution is skewed to the left (negative) or to the right (positive) of the theoretical center of gravity (Figs. 12-7 and 12-8). The extent of the negative and positive directions is measured by standard deviations.

FREQUENCY DISTRIBUTIONS

A beginning point for the researcher in identifying the character of a curve is to inspect the nature of the values (numbers) that are incorporated in it. This may be accomplished by tallying a frequency distribution of those values (numbers) in either ascending or descending order. Thus, a frequency distribution is the classification of numbers that are or are not recurrent. This organization is developed so that data can be summarized from their original disorganization.

The form that the frequency classification takes is based on the research question being asked. For example, suppose a public health nurse becomes aware of the questionable nutritional status because of

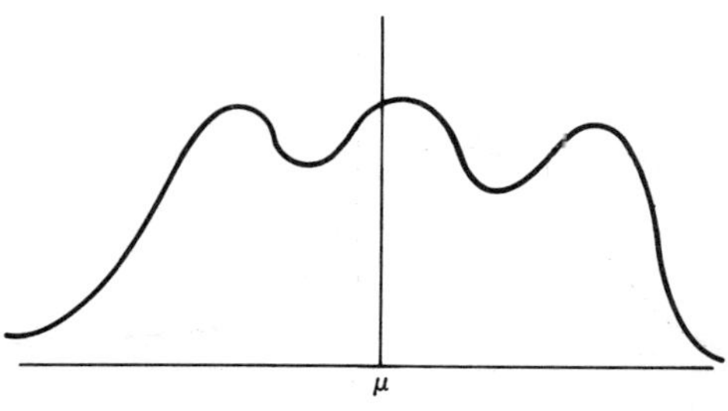

Figure 12-6. Trimodal curve.

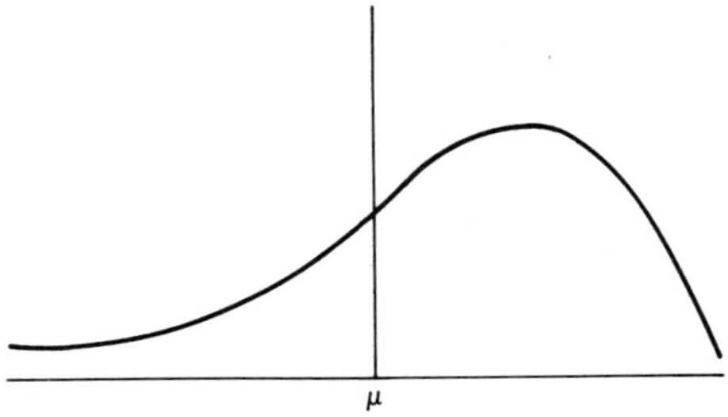

Figure 12-7. Distribution curve skewed to left (negative).

obesity of some of the families in her district. She may wonder if there is a relationship between the age of the food preparer and the amount of apparent obesity in the family. She uses questionnaires to gather data from 10 people who prepare meals, carefully collecting their cooking habits as well as their ages.

A first step in organizing the data on the 10 questionnaires is to develop a frequency distribution of the ages of the respondents (Table 12-4). This example gives the ages in ascending order. The ages would be tallied in the following manner:

1. Group the questionnaires by age and note that the age spread is from 18 to 64 years, with one person (f) listed for each age. A table is described by its rows and colums, with the rows on the horizontal axis and columns on the vertical axis. The column headings are ages (X) and frequencies (f). The table title should be descriptive of the table so that the reader can quickly determine the topic of its contents.

2. Determine the frequency of occurrence of each age (f) so that Table 12-4 now becomes more refined, as shown in Table 12-5. The data may be grouped or ungrouped. These data of ages are ungrouped.

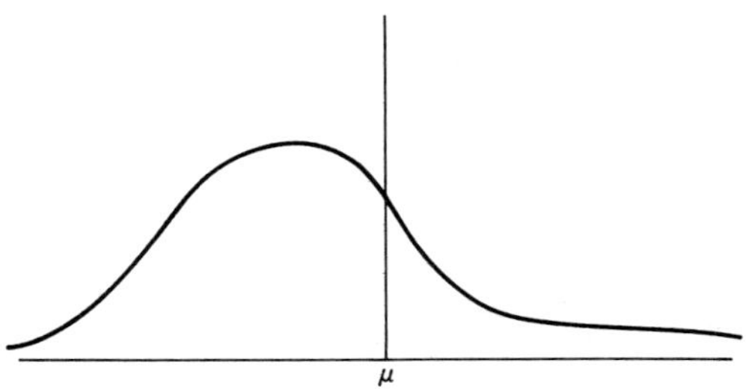

Figure 12-8. Distribution curve skewed to right (positive).

Table 12-4. Age of Ten Respondents in Obesity Study

Age in Years (X)	*Frequency (f)*
18	1
22	1
35	1
52	1
52	1
60	1
63	1
63	1
63	1
64	1
	10

If the researcher were analyzing data of 100 ages, for example, she might group her data for ease of handling. In this instance she would inspect the ages and determine whether or not they fall into natural groups. For example, in the 100 ages she may see that most of the respondents are between 30 and 75 years of age. In this instance, she may choose to group the ages by 10-year intervals, that is, 31–40; 41–50; 51–60; 61–70; 71–80, always being careful not to overlap the intervals. Should an overlap occur, groups then would include the same person in more than one age. For example, of the 100 respondents, 70 may be between 61 and 70 years of age. This may not matter, but in our example, in which the nurse would be specifically concerned about

Table 12-5. Age of Ten Respondents in Obesity Study

Age in Years (X)	*Frequency (f)*
18	1
22	1
35	1
52	2
60	1
63	3
64	1
	10

the age of the person and her food preparation habits, she would want the ages to be more clearly defined. How many people are 62, 63, 64, and so on? Is there a relationship between cooking habits and older people? Clearly, whether or not data are grouped and, if so, how they are grouped, are dependent on the research question and hypotheses to be tested.

Another way of exploring data could be by the stem and leaf method (Tukey, 1970). Tukey suggests that exploratory data analysis is detective work of a numerical, counting, or graphical nature. Numbers should be handled easily and effectively. Techniques should be kept simple so long as they work well and reveal the unexpected surprises. Details should be emphasized only when they make a difference. Otherwise they should be suppressed.

The stem and leaf method meets these criteria (Fig. 12-9). It is a way of displaying data without losing the actual numbers as they are lost in grouped data. The first part of a number (each line) is the stem, and the leaf is each piece of information in the stem. For example, if we had 50 ages from 30 to 80 years to describe, the stem columns would include 3, 4, 5, 6, 7, and 8. The leaves would indicate the specific ages of people who are in the 30-year range, 40-year range, and so on. Clearly more people are 66 years old than any other age.

The technique is useful for several reasons. First, as seen in Figure 12-9, it indicates the nature of the curve. Turned on its vertical axis, it becomes a histogram. A histogram is a bar graph giving a pictorial display of the data. It is developed by organizing them into classes. The bars show how many numbers are in the various classes. The stem and

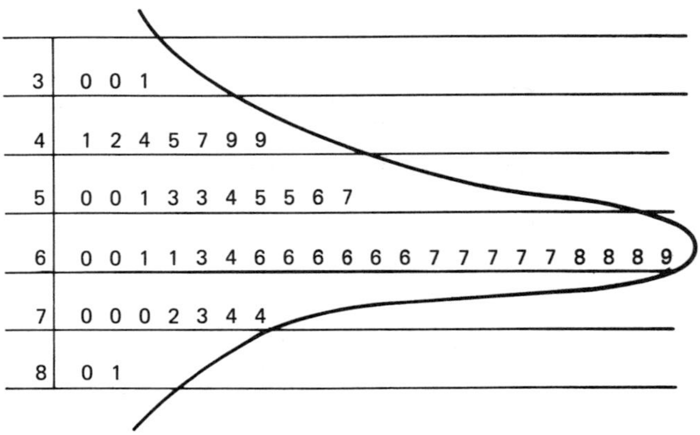

Figure 12-9. Stem and leaf.

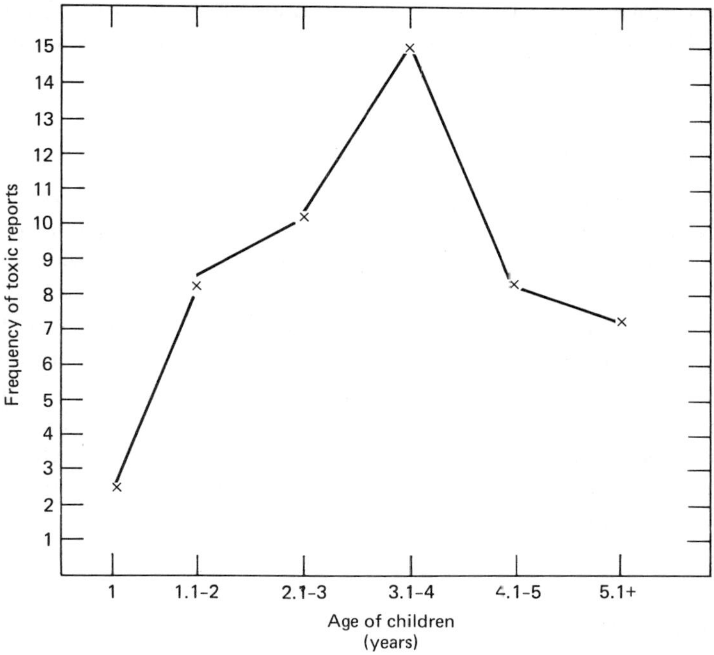

Figure 12-10. Frequency of toxic reports for children in the State Department Well Child Clinic, by age.

leaf process also identifies the "(1) appearances of separation into groups, (2) unsymmetric trailing off, going further in one direction than another, (3) unexpected popular or unpopular values, (4) about where these values are 'centered,' and (5) about how widely values spread" (Tukey, 1970, pp. 1–27).

By using the stem and leaf method, the researcher has a quick indication of the shape of the distribution. A more precise method to gain this information would be to plot the data on graph paper. For example, if a researcher were questioning the increased number of toxic materials ingested by children in a particular health department well-child clinic, she might wonder if the age of the children could be related to the accidents. She could review 50 charts of the children to determine their ages. Plotted data may indicate a curve such as depicted in Figure 12-10. This graph tells us that the curve is unimodal and skewed to the left or negative (see Fig. 12-8). The researcher may determine that children in the younger age groups are at apparent risk of poison ingestion. In addition, the researcher may wonder if reporting practices explain this distribution. Are the younger children really ingesting more toxic materials or are nurses more careful in reporting their activities? These questions would require further investigation.

SUMMARY

This chapter has presented several basic ideas related to descriptive statistics. Descriptive data must be systematic and objective so that the researcher is able to make some general statements about the study group variables.

Special focus has been on measures of central tendency, including the mean, mode, and median. Measures of dispersion, including the standard deviation, variance, and range were presented. The normal distribution curve, including the standardized Z score, and frequency distributions, with special emphasis on the stem and leaf method, were explained. Examples were included to illustrate their uses, methods of calculation, and importance.

BIBLIOGRAPHY

Blalock, H. M., Jr. *Social Statistics,* 2nd edition. New York: McGraw-Hill, 1972.

Dixon, W. J., & Massey, F. J. Jr. *Introduction to Statistical Analysis,* 3rd edition. New York: McGraw-Hill, 1969.

Duncan, R. C., Knapp, R. G., & Miller, M. C. *Introductory Biostatistics for the Health Sciences.* New York: John Wiley & Sons, 1977.

Snedecor, G. W., & Cochran, W. G. *Statistical Methods,* 6th edition. Ames, Iowa: The Iowa State University Press, 1972, p. 51.

Tukey, J. W. *Exploring Data Analysis,* Vol. I. Reading, Massachusetts: Addison-Wesley, 1970.

13
Parametric and Nonparametric Statistics

Parametric and nonparametric (NP) statistics are those tools that allow the researcher to analyze sample or study group data. This chapter focuses on the use of these tools in analysis and interpretation. Many nursing studies include a relatively small number of research subjects. When it has been shown that the sample does not represent the population from which it was drawn and that it may not be possible to make inferences about the population, nonparametric statistics may be used (see Chap. 9). A presentation of two nonparametric statistical tests is included.

Specific examples of statistical tests frequently used in nursing research are presented along with illustrations of procedures for their calculations. In Chapter 12 methods for describing samples were presented. This chapter introduces some statistical tests used in analyzing data so that generalizations about the population or summary statements about the study group can be made.

PARAMETRIC STATISTICS

"Parameters are the fixed values that refer to population and generally are unknown" (Blalock, 1972, p. 110). As can be seen in Chapter 12, the parameters of a normal distribution are the mean (μ) and the variance (σ^2). If observations are drawn at random and are normally distributed, they are ideal and can be used in statistical tests. It is important to ascertain that the assumptions underlying the statistical test are satisfied before using the test. Therefore, a parametric statistical test is one whose underlying assumptions—model—specify certain conditions about the distribution of the population from which the research sample was drawn (Dixon and Massey, 1969). However, the researcher may not know how representative the sample actually is of that population. Employing the appropriate statistical test will help to clarify this question.

Parametric statistics allow the researcher to determine whether it is possible to make generalized statements—inferences—about the sample. This is accomplished by providing a means for determining the extent of differences between the sample and the population from which it was drawn. The focus is on the population and how the sample represents it. It is important to compare some quantitative difference against the natural variation that exists in the data. The testing of hypotheses is based on these differences. Therefore, the major use of parametric statistics is to provide an indication of the extent and direction of the differences between the population values and the sample values.

t Test

One of the most frequently used parametric statistical tests in nursing research is the *t* test. This test was first derived in 1908 by W. S. Gosset, an Irish brewery employee. He published his work under the pseudonym Student, and often this test is referred to as the Student *t* test (Johnson, 1976). This text will refer to it as the *t* test.

The *t* test is used for comparing the mean of the sample with the mean of the population from which the sample was drawn. The *t* test is also used for making inferences about the means of two samples that are either independent or paired. The two independent samples may be of equal or unequal sizes. Obviously, the paired samples are of equal sizes.

The size of the sample is an important element in the use of the *t* test. The test is most useful when the sample size (N) is equal to or less than ($\leq$) 30 observations. Mathematically, it has been shown that the standard deviation (SD) calculated from any sample is an underestimation of the standard deviation of the universe. Because of this fact, the denominator is adjusted in the standard deviation formula by subtracting 1 from the number of observations ($n - 1$) so that the variance will approximate more closely the population variance. This adjustment ($n - 1$) gives the degree of freedom (df) (Bancroft, 1967). Degrees of freedom "reflect the number of observations that are free to vary after certain restrictions are placed on the data" (Siegel, 1956, p. 44). Knowing the number of degrees of freedom in a sample is essential for the use of a *t* table.

A t table contains a different t distribution for every sample size. Each is like a normal distribution in that it centers on zero and is symmetrical. However, as the sample size increases, the distribution of the t curve more closely approximates the normal curve—the Z distribution (see Appendix Table B). To use this table, the sample size, number of degrees of freedom, and t value must be known. The table will indicate the level of significance of the calculated t value.

In order to use the t test appropriately, we must be assured that certain assumptions are met. These include

1. Distribution of variables in the population from which the sample was drawn are normal.
2. Samples have equal variances if the two-sample t test is used.
3. Samples were drawn by random sampling.

The formula for the single sample t test, in which we are to compare the sample with the hypothesized mean (μ) population, is

$$\underset{n-1}{t} = \frac{\bar{X} - \mu}{s/\sqrt{n}}$$

where n is sample size, $n - 1$ is the degree of freedom, $\bar{X}$ is the sample mean, μ is the population mean, and $s/\sqrt{n}$ is the estimate of the standard error of the mean $\bar{X}$ (estimation of the SD of the sampling distribution).

To illustrate the use of the t test with one sample, suppose we want to evaluate the success of a child immunization program using a random sample of 25 public health agencies in one state. The percent (%) of attendance (success) of child immunization programs in the agencies (population) has been kept. A standard was set that the mean success for all immunization programs ought to be at least 60%. In the sample ($N = 25$) the mean is calculated to be 52% and the standard deviation is 12%. The null hypothesis is that there is no statistical difference between the sample mean and the population mean. The question is asked: Is the level of performance in the population programs significantly below the standard expected? The hypotheses are σ = unknown, $\bar{X} = 52\%$, $\mu = 60\%$, $df = 25 - 1 = 24$. The rejection level is set at $P \leqslant .05$. After determining the rejection level, we consult the t table and note where the t value would have to lie in order for the hypothesis to be accepted or rejected. This table gives the values that are in the "tails" of the distribution. We note that we need a t value of 1.7109 (one tail) or *larger* to get a significant difference between the two means.

Next, we fit our values into the t formula and find

$$t = \frac{51 - 60}{12/\sqrt{25}} = \frac{-9}{12/\sqrt{25}} = \frac{-9}{2.40} = -3.75$$

We said that a t value $\geqslant$ 1.7109 would be within the critical (rejection) region (5%). Our result is -3.75; therefore we reject the hypothesis that $\mu = 60$ and conclude (with a 5% risk of error) that the actual performance of the immunization programs is below the standard expected. A t value of -3.75 is greater than the probability of .005.

Suppose the researcher wants to compare the means of two independent samples of unequal sizes. For example, in comparing the weight gains of obese adolescents under two diets, the null hypothesis is that there is no significant difference between the two sample means. The t test is used to determine whether the means of the two samples are significantly different from the population mean. In other words, theoretically, do the samples come from the same population? The research hypothesis is: Adolescents on high protein diets gain significantly more weight than do adolescents on low protein diets. The significance level is set at $P < .05$, one-tailed. One tail of the t distribution is used because the hypothesis states one direction, that is, *more weight.* Table 13-1 gives the data showing weight gains measured in pounds under the two diets.

When there are two samples, there are two variances (s_1^2 and s_2^2). In the example of the obese adolescents, the two variances are $s_1^2 = 2497.33$ and $s_2^2 = 2138.75$. In order to use the variances for the t test, we must pool them to get the average (Snedecor and Cochran, 1967). The formula used for the pooled variance ($s^2{}_p$) is

$$s_p{}^2 = \frac{\Sigma x_1^2 + x_2^2}{(N_1 - 1) + (N_2 - 1)} = \frac{\overset{s_1^2}{2497.33} + \overset{s_2^2}{2138.75}}{5 + 3}$$

$$= \frac{4636.08}{8}$$

$$= 579.51 \qquad df = 8$$

Table 13-1. Weight (lb) of 10 Children on Protein Diets

	X *High-Protein Diet*	Y *Low-Protein Diet*
	134	70
	146	118
	104	101
	119	132
	124	—
	83	—
Totals	710	421

$N = 6$

$\overline{X} = \frac{710}{6} = 118.33$

$\Sigma X^2 = 134^2 + 146^2 + 104^2 + 119^2 + 124^2 + 83^2 = 86{,}514$

$(\Sigma X)^2/N = \frac{(710)^2}{6} = 84{,}016.67$

$\Sigma X = 86{,}514 - 84{,}016.67$
$= 2497.33$

$df = 6 - 1 = 5$

$N = 4$

$\overline{X} = 105.25$

$\Sigma Y^2 = 46{,}449$

$(\Sigma Y)^2/N =$
$44{,}310.25$

$46{,}449 - 44{,}310.25 = 2138.75$

$df = 4 - 1 = 3$

Finally, we need to calculate the standard error of the difference of the means of the two samples. The standard error is the standard deviation of the sampling distribution and is calculated as

$$S_{\overline{X}_1} - \overline{X}_2 = \sqrt{s_p^2 \frac{(N_1 + N_2)}{N_1 N_2}} = \sqrt{579.51 \times \frac{6 + 4}{(6)(4)}}$$
$$= \sqrt{579.51(.417)} = 15.55 \text{ lb}$$

With these calculations completed, we apply the t test to determine if the means of the two samples are significantly different.

$$t = \frac{(\overline{X}_1 - \overline{X}_2)}{S/\sqrt{\overline{X}_1 - \overline{X}_2}} = \frac{(118.33 - 105.25)}{11.55}$$
$$= .84 \qquad df = 8$$

After consulting the t table (see Appendix Table B), we determine that the t value at $P < .05$ (one-tailed) is 1.86. Our t value, .84, is much lower than the table value. Remember that we need a t value that is equal to or greater than the value in the t table.

With this information we can say that there appears to be no significant difference in the weight gains between the two groups due to different protein diets. We could accept the null hypothesis of no difference and reject any stated differences. In other words, the amount of protein eaten by the children in the two groups apparently has no effect on their weight gains.

Regression and Correlation

This section presents a brief discussion of regression and correlation analyses and their underlying assumptions, and it gives examples of their uses. Both statistics are used to examine the relationship between two variables. It is beyond the scope of this text to present detailed information on the derivations and calculations of regression. Also, this text will not discuss Analysis of Variance (ANOVA). It is suggested that the student consult a statistical textbook, such as Draper and Smith (1966), for this information. Special attention is given to correlation methods.

Regression

Regression is the type of analysis that examines the *effect* that one variable has on another. We want to determine the effect that the independent variable (X) has on the dependent variable (Y). Specifically, regression is used to learn if Y depends on X and to predict Y from X. Regression answers such as: Does educational level have an effect on income? Does age have an effect on blood pressure levels? We are looking for the regression of educational levels (X) on income (Y) or age (X) on blood pressure (Y). The distribution of the X variables is fixed; in other words, the X's are considered constants, and each of the Y variables will have a distribution. Similarly, there will be a blood pressure for individuals by age, and each distribution will have a mean and variance. The straight line, that is, the path of the means of the Y variables, blood pressure, for X age, is found using the simple linear regression equation.

The assumptions underlying the simplest regression models are

1. Regression equation has a linear form.
2. Distribution of Y values is normal for each X value.

3. Variance of Y distribution is the same for each X value (Blalock, 1972).

The regression equation is

$$Y = \alpha + BX$$

where Y is the dependent variable, α is that point where the line intercepts the Y axis, B is the constant slope term, and X is the independent variable. (In mathematics this is called a function; that is, Y is a function of X.) Using the regression formula, the unique straight line is found where the sum of squares of the deviations of the observed Y from the predicted $\alpha + bx$ are at a minimum.

Once data are plotted on the X axis, the regression equation is used to fit the line in order to determine the nature of the relationship. For example, suppose a researcher observed that some hospital nurses are promoted more quickly than others and wonders if this may be related to their educational levels. The goal is to predict the effects of annual income of nurses on their educational levels in this hypothetical setting. Through the appropriate ethics review committee, permission is granted to review the full-time nursing personnel records regarding their salary and education level (type of diploma: associate arts, baccalaureate, master's). Findings may resemble those shown in Figure 13-1. This

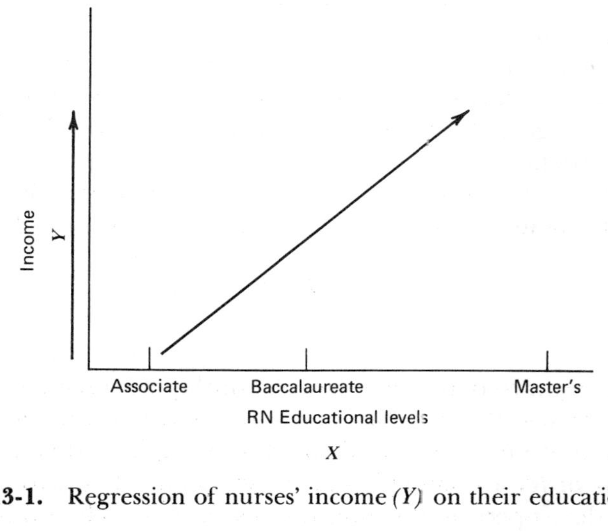

Figure 13-1. Regression of nurses' income (Y) on their education levels.

figure shows the regression of income on education. For this hospital setting, it can be said that nurses with higher education earn higher salaries. Presumably, nurses with master's degrees would hold more highly paid positions than would nurses with associate arts degrees. Regression analysis permits these statements to be made.

Correlation

Correlation is similar to regression in that it is a technique of inference. It, too, measures the degree of linear association between two possibly related variables. However, if the relationship is weak, there is no point in trying to predict Y from X. The *strength* of the relationship is determined with correlation. It is possible to say that changes of values in one variable are associated with the changes of values in another variable. Note that both X and Y are considered variables now as opposed to only Y being a variable in regression. The changes of values, in correlation, are accomplished entirely by observation. For example, the researcher would observe one person on one variable and the same person on a second variable and note the strength of that relationship. Correlation values indicate the strength of an association and in no way may alter or change the form of that relationship. Also, if cause-and-effect relationships exist between the two variables under study, they cannot be detected using the correlation statistic.

The correlation coefficient was introduced by Karl Pearson and is often referred to as the Pearson product-moment correlation rho (r) (Blalock, 1972). It is easily interpreted and ranges from -1.0 to $+1.0$. A relationship initially may be inspected by displaying it in a scatter diagram, where the X values are plotted in relation to the Y values. This provides a visual impression of the strength and direction of the relationship. Figure 13-2 shows the various possible relationships between two variables.

The Pearson product-moment correlation coefficient r is the statistic used to determine the extent of the linear relationship (-1.0 – $+1.0$).

$$r = \frac{\Sigma^{z}X^{z}Y}{N}$$

Suppose we want to determine the relationship between two sets of test scores, where X = the first half of the test and Y = the second half of the test. Four students are used for this example, rather than a large number, in order to simplify the presentation. The two sets of test scores are developed by dividing the test in half. The odd-numbered items could comprise one group, and the even-numbered items the

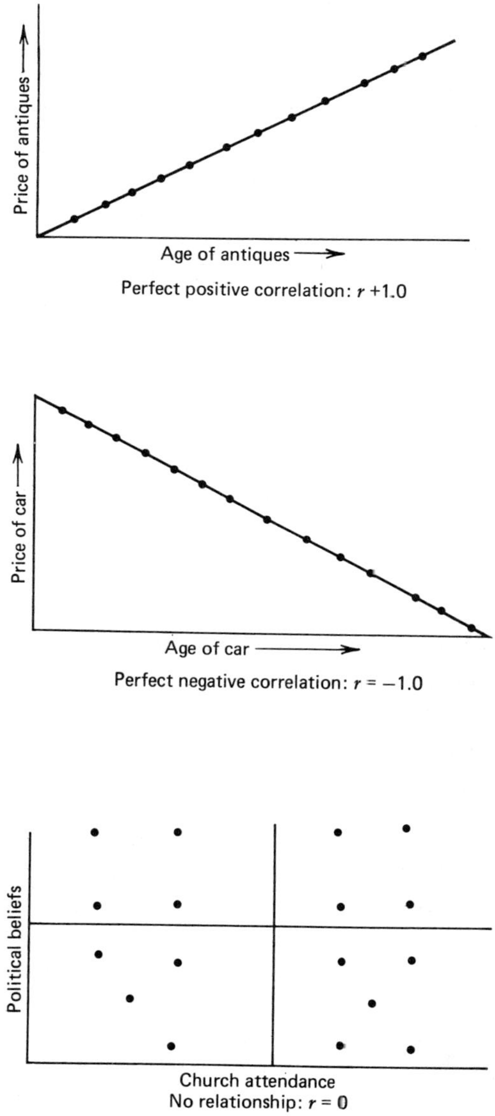

Figure 13-2. Correlation relationships between two variables.

other. A comparison of the performance of each group of test items is made.

In plotting the scores we find a nearly perfect negative correlation (Fig. 13-3).

The calculations are shown in Table 13-2.

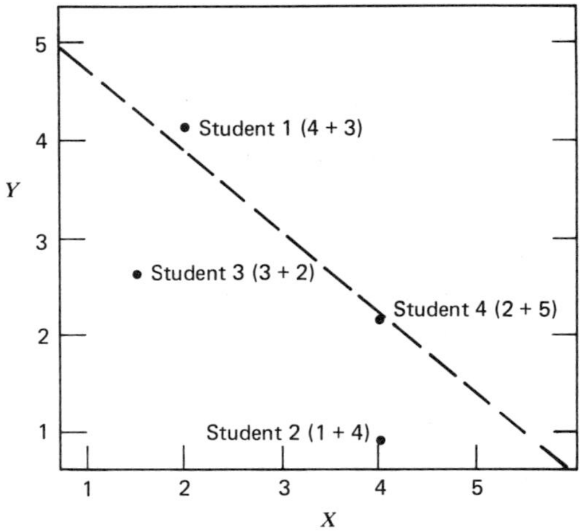

Figure 13-3. Diagram of ODD/EVEN test scores for four students.

The procedure can be summarized as follows:

1. List all the X and Y scores for each person.
2. Convert them to Z scores to approximate a normal distribution.
3. Multiply each subject's $Z_x Z_y$ score.
4. Sum these figures.
5. Divide by the number of subjects.

Consulting Table 13-3, we can interpret the figures as follows: With an r value of $-.603$, we can say that as the X scores improved, the Y scores dropped. Students did better on the first half of the test than on the second half. This finding would lead us to inspect our test for its lack of reliability and consider its reconstruction. The reliability of a test in which one half appears easier than its other half would be questionable. Chapter 8 offers a full discussion of reliability.

It is possible to be more specific about the interpretation of this r value by squaring it; in this case, $r^2 = .36$. Squaring eliminates the negative numbers and puts the values on a scale that has a lower limit of zero and thus measures the strength of the relationship. It is now known that about ⅓ (36%) of the variance in the Y scores is associated with the X scores and that about 64% of the variance is not explained through its relation with X. Hence, r^2 describes the proportion of the variance in Y that can be attributed to its linear correlation with X. In other words, $1 - r^2$ is the proportion of the variance of Y that is free

Table 13-2. Relationship of Test Scores for Four Students Using Pearson Product-Moment Correlation

Student	*X Score*	X^2	$\frac{X - \bar{X}}{SD}$	=	*ZX*
1	3	9	$\frac{3 - 3.5}{1.12}$	=	−.45
2	4	16	$\frac{4 - 3.5}{1.12}$	=	.45
3	2	4	$\frac{2 - 3.5}{1.12}$	=	−1.34
4	5	25	$\frac{5 - 3.5}{1.12}$	=	1.34
	$\Sigma X = 14$	$\Sigma X^2 = 54$			

$X = \frac{14}{4} = 3.5$

$X^2 = 12.25$

$SD = \sqrt{\frac{\Sigma X^2}{N} - \bar{X}^2} = \sqrt{\frac{54}{4} - 12.25}$

$SD_X = 1.12$

$ZX = \frac{X - \bar{X}}{SD}$

Student	*Y Score*	Y^2	$\frac{Y - \bar{Y}}{SD}$	=	*ZY*	$Z_X Z_Y$
1	4	16	$\frac{4 - 2.5}{1.12}$	=	1.34	−.603
2	1	1	$\frac{1 - 2.5}{1.12}$	=	−1.34	−.603
3	3	9	$\frac{3 - 2.5}{1.12}$	=	.45	−.603
4	2	4	$\frac{2 - 2.5}{1.12}$	=	.45	−.603
	$ZY = 10$	$ZY^2 = 30$				$\Sigma Z_X Z_Y = -\ 2.412$

$\bar{Y} = \frac{10}{4} = 2.5$

$\bar{Y}^2 = 6.28$

$SD = \sqrt{\frac{30}{4 - 6.25}}$

$= 1.12$

$ZY = \frac{Y - \bar{Y}}{SD}$

$r = \frac{-2.412}{4}$

$r = -.603$

from X, that is, not explained by X. As r increases, $1 - r^2$ decreases. For example, given an $r \pm .1$, r^2 would be .01 and $1 - r^2$ would be .99. This value indicates to the researcher that 99% of the variation between the X and Y scores cannot be explained by their relationship. If given an $r \pm .9$ and r^2 of .81, then $1 - r^2$ would be .19. Similarly, 19% of the variation between the X and Y scores cannot be explained. As the r value gets closer to 1, it is known that more of the variance in the Y scores is associated with the X scores and less variance is unexplained.

As can be seen, this process indicates to the educator the amount of explained variation between the X and Y variables. If there were a large amount of unexplained variation, the educator may wish to consider the reliability of the test itself and the process used in the test administration. Evidence of causality, that is, that X causes variation in Y, cannot be shown. However, the Y scores could be predicted from the X scores using the regression equation $Y = \alpha + Bx + e$ (error).

NONPARAMETRIC STATISTICS

Recall that parametric statistics were defined as referring to populations with normal distributions. When we make inferences about the population from which the sample was drawn, our statistical assumptions make that possible.

Nonparametric statistics refer to a sample in which there may be no assumptions made about the population from which the sample was drawn. We usually use these statistics with small samples, N less than 30. If the samples are larger than 30, we may be able to fit the distribution of data to the normal curve and use parametric statistics.

Although there are many nonparametric statistical tests, this section presents examples of the two that are more commonly used in nursing research. Specifically, these include Spearman's rho (ρ) and chi square (χ^2). Additional procedures may be found in nonparametric statistics texts such as Siegel (1956) and Hollander and Wolfe (1973).

Spearman's Rank-Order Correlation Coefficient

The rank-order correlation coefficient test developed by Spearman in 1904 is used for a nonnormal population that has ranks and orders (Siegel, 1956). It is an ordinal scale correlation and has no notion of linearity. The rankings of two sets of data are compared to determine their relationship. This relationship may either increase or decrease; that is, the greater the X value the greater or lesser the Y value. The extent of that relationship, is indicated by ρ. It is an estimate from -1 to $+1$ and is used when there is a small N. (See Appendix Table C.)

Suppose we want to determine if the number of study hours per week for certain nursing students is related to their place of residence. We have 12 senior nursing students who have spent six months living in the nurses' residence and six months living in their homes. They switched their housing during their senior year of nursing school. The reasons for their relocation are unimportant to this example. Our null hypothesis is that there is no difference in the amount of study time (hours) per week of the nursing students between the two locations. We set the $P < .01$.

The Spearman formula is

$$\rho = 1 - \frac{6\Sigma d^2}{N^3 - N}$$

where d is the difference between the ranks (X and Y), N is the number of subjects, and Σd^2 is the sum of the squared differences.

The rank of the observations is determined by inspecting the array of the values and assigning the number 1 to the smallest number of hours and 12 to the largest number of hours. In this example we have several ties. For instance, we have two subjects in the dormitory setting who spent 10.2 hours in study time. When such ties occur, we take the average of the rankings so that 10.2 does not become numbers 1 and 2 in the ranking. Rather the two ranks are averaged, and each value is assigned the rank of 1.5. This process is followed for all tied rankings (Table 13-3).

In this statistic actual differences between the ranks are squared and summed. A ρ value of $+1$ would indicate perfect agreement in the rankings, -1 would indicate perfect disagreement, and a ρ of 0 would indicate no relationship.

The calculation for ρ in Table 13-3 is

$$P = 1 - \frac{6(42.00)}{1728 - 12} = 1 - \frac{252.00}{1716.00} = 1 - .147$$

$$\rho = .853$$

$$P < .001$$

When we have a ρ of .853 ($P < .001$), we reject our null hypothesis. Apparently there is a difference in the amount of study time spent by

Table 13-3. Effects of Housing Location on Study Habits of 12 Nursing Students

Subject	*Dorm Hours/Week* *Y*	*Rank* *X*	*Home Hours/Week* *Y*	*Rank* *X*	*d*	d^2
1	10.4	4	7.4	5	−1	1
2	10.8	8.5	7.6	7	1.5	2.25
3	11.1	10	7.9	11	−1	1
4	10.2	1.5	7.2	2.5	−1	1
5	10.3	3	7.4	5	−2	4
6	10.2	1.5	7.1	1	0.5	.25
7	10.7	7	7.4	5	2	4
8	10.5	5	7.2	2.5	2.5	6.25
9	10.8	8.5	7.8	9.5	−1	1
10	11.2	11	7.7	8	3	9
11	10.6	6	7.8	9.5	−3.5	12.25
12	11.4	12	8.3	12	0	0
					$\sum d^2$ =	42.00

nurses in the two settings. Nurses living in a dormitory spend more hours studying per week than when they live at home.

The conclusions that we reach about this finding would depend on our specific research question. For instance, were we attempting to show need for less dormitory space, smaller rooms, one person per room allocation? If this were so, we would reconsider these needs and perhaps conclude that dormitory nurses tended to aid each other in their study habits and thus spend more time in group studying. We might also be interested in comparing the difference in test results of students in the two settings to determine whether the hours devoted to studying had a positive effect on their grades. Clearly, this question would have to be carefully defined before any data collection was undertaken.

Chi Square

The chi square (χ^2) test is a general test used when we want to determine if the observed frequencies of values collected in our study differ from those that we may expect to occur as a result of chance. Many nonparametric statistical tests measure the *existence* of such relationships between two variables. However, chi square measures the *strength* of the relationship between two or more variables. It can be used when we want to compare observed sample values (observations, subjects, etc.) with a theoretical frequency distribution that is normal. This is called the "goodness of fit" test, and it measures how well the values in our sample fit the distribution. Also, chi square is used as a measure of the strength of association between two or more independent groups. This measure is the one more often used in nursing research and will be the focus of this presentation. We will illustrate the use of χ^2 for two independent samples using artifical data.

To use the χ^2 test, we must not have any zeros in the expected frequency cells, and these cells cannot have less than 1–5 cases in more than 20% of them. If these frequencies occur, we must either collapse the cells in the tables to adjust for the presence of zeros or use Yates' correction for continuity. This text will not present these methods. The interested reader is referred to Fleiss (1973, Chaps. 2 and 10) for a presentation of these procedures. These problems can be avoided if the researcher plans in advance and collects large samples.

Assumptions underlying the use of χ^2 are

1. Two or more nominal scales of measurement are used.
2. Samples are randomly drawn and are independent.

Suppose we are interested in inspecting the number of nonhealth-related activities that nurses and physicians engage in for relaxation during their last year of education. We determine that recreational activities can be categorized as 1) sport that involves teams (baseball, volleyball, etc.) and 2) quiet activities that involve one or two people (cards, backgammon, etc.). We draw a sample that consists of 30 RNs and 30 MDs. These people are students in their last year of professional education. Our null hypothesis (H_0) is: There is no difference in modes of relaxation between nurses and physicians during the last year of their educational programs. We will accept this H_0 at $P < .05$ and it is tested with:

$$\chi^2 = \Sigma \frac{(O - E)^2}{E}$$

where O is observed frequencies and E is expected frequencies. The χ^2 values are presented in Appendix Table D.

In order to calculate the χ^2 test, we must compute the degrees of freedom (df) that are involved. This calculation is based on the number of rows $(r - 1)$ and columns $(k - 1)$ that the data comprise. Table 13-4 is a 2×2 contingency table. It has 2 rows and 2 columns, so the $df = (2 - 1)(2 - 1) = 1$. This tells us that we would need to calculate the

Table 13-4. Activities of RNs and MDs During Last Year of Professional Education

	Quiet		*Sports*		
	Observed	*Expected*	*Observed*	*Expected*	*Totals*
RNs	20	17.5	10	12.5	30
MDs	15	17.5	15	12.5	30
Totals	35	35	25	25	60

$$\chi^2 = \sum \frac{(20 - 17.5)^2}{17.5} + \frac{(15 - 17.5)^2}{17.5} + \frac{(10 - 12.5)^2}{12.5} + \frac{(15 - 12.5)^2}{12.5}$$

$$= .357 + .357 + .5 + .5$$

$$= 1.714 \quad df = 1 \quad P < .10$$

value for one cell once we had ascertained the values for the other rows and columns. If we were using a 2×3 table, the *df* would be $(2 - 1)(3 - 1) = 2$, and so forth. There is a different χ^2 distribution for each *df*. (See Appendix Table D.)

Calculation of the expected values is based on the marginal totals. In our table the expected value for nurses in quiet activities is determined by

$$^{35}/_{60} \times 30 = 17.5$$

$$35 - 17.5 = 17.5 = E \text{ value for RNs}$$

This same process is followed for the expected value cells for physicians. Thus we get

$$^{25}/_{60} \times 30 = 12.5$$

$$25 - 12.5 = 12.5 = E \text{ value for MDs}$$

Now that we have our table complete and have determined the *df*, we can proceed with the χ^2 calculation (see Table 13-4).

These data show that there is no significant difference between the observed and expected frequencies in the two groups. The null hypothesis holds, and it is accepted. If we had set the P value $< .01$, the difference would have been significant. In that event we would inspect the data and see which cell had the highest frequency. This would have told us the most preferred activity and by which group it was preferred.

SUMMARY

This chapter has presented an overview of the use of parametric and nonparametric statistics in nursing research. Examples of the *t* test, Pearson Product-Moment Correlation Coefficient, chi square, and Spearman's rho were presented indicating their underlying assumptions, uses, and methods of calculations. In all examples the questions were hypothetical, and the data were artificial. The chapter was meant to serve as a beginning point in the statistical analysis of collected data. The reader is urged to consult more advanced statistics textbooks for further information on any of the presented topics.

BIBLIOGRAPHY

Bancroft, H. *Introduction to Biostatistics.* New York: Harper & Row, 1967.

Blalock, A. M., Jr. *Social Statistics,* 6th edition. New York: McGraw-Hill, 1972.

Dixon, W. J., & Massey, F. J., Jr. *Introduction to Statistical Analysis,* 3rd edition. New York: McGraw-Hill, 1969.

Draper, N. R., & Smith, H. *Applied Regression Analysis.* New York: John Wiley & Sons, 1976.

Fleiss, J. L. *Statistical Methods for Rates and Proportions.* New York: John Wiley & Sons, 1973.

Hollander, W., & Wolfe, D. A. *Non-Parametric Statistical Methods.* New York: John Wiley & Sons, 1976.

Johnson, R. *Elementary Statistics,* 2nd edition. North Scituate, Massachusetts: Duxbury Press, 1976.

Snedecor, G. W., & Cochran, W. G. *Statistical Methods* 6th edition. Ames, Iowa: Iowa State University Press, 1972.

Siegel, S. *Non-Parametric Statistics For The Behavioral Sciences.* New York: McGraw-Hill, 1956.

14
Presentation and Interpretation of Findings

Caroline M. White

Presentation and interpretation of findings are critical steps in the research process. The care that was taken to review the literature, identify a theoretical framework, design the study, and conduct it now pays off in terms of findings to be shared. The clarity with which findings are presented and the astuteness and honesty of the investigator as the findings are interpreted influence the extent to which the study is accorded recognition as a contribution to the science of nursing.

Findings are the information that was gained as a result of the research effort. Findings refer to the relationships that are discovered among the study variables; they are the results of the analysis. Findings also refer to descriptions of the study sample. Serendipitous findings are those insights or observations that were made in conjunction with the process of conducting the study; they arise from the study but may not relate to the specific purpose of the study.

Interpretations are the inferences that emerge from the study findings, the explanations that are offered to justify why the findings indicated the relationships they did, and the implications for further research, practice, and theory that might be attributed to the findings.

This chapter discusses methods for presenting study findings and questions to be considered for their accurate interpretation.

PRESENTATION OF FINDINGS: WHAT AND HOW

The researcher must consider two questions with respect to presentation of findings: What to present? How to present it? These are eternal questions; they arise each time a person wants to convey information to another person, and, no matter how experienced the presenter, there are dilemmas. When research results are to be reported, the concerns are the same as those that operate when there is need for one student to communicate with another or to an instructor about the progress of a patient. The factors to be considered are purpose of the communication; audience for the communication; and limits imposed by others with respect to the length of the communication, topics to be covered, and acceptable or feasible means to convey the information.

Purpose of the Research Report

Presentations of research may be designed to convey a complete report of the study (literature review, theoretical framework, research questions or hypotheses, methodology, findings, interpretations, and recommendations). In this case, it is appropriate to follow a published format for presentations of research. A complete report of the research should allow people hearing or reading the report to understand how the investigator arrived at questions for study, how the study was conducted, and the answers to the study questions. A good way to check on the completeness of a formal report is to evaluate it using a published article that discusses how to critique a research report. This evaluation can show the extent to which major issues and points have been covered in the report being prepared. The reader is directed to Chapter 15 of this book and Ward (1979) for further discussion.

Sometimes findings of a study are presented without the extensive background information contained in a formal report of research. In this case, it is appropriate to design the presentation by giving consideration to the extent of precision and detail required for understanding, for giving a basis for decision, or for describing the elements studied. It is usually advisable to consult with a more experienced person so that an appropriate presentation is designed.

Audience

Some audiences are more sophisticated than others, and this sophistication should be considered as the presentation of findings is designed. The use of words, the complexity of sentences, the use of visual aids, and the actual content of the presentation all must be designed so that the audience can comprehend the presentation.

The nature of the audience; their level of education; their degree of familiarity with the topic, with the particular research procedures, and with the techniques of analysis employed; and their possible purpose(s) in reading or receiving the report should guide the selection of material for presentation. Often it is possible to learn in advance of the presentation the interests and sophistication of the audience. The effort taken to do this is usually worthwhile for the reception both of the presenter and that of the findings, and the value the audience may come to place on the research process itself.

Limits Imposed By Others

The presenter of findings may have to work within constraints imposed by others. These arise from limitations of time, number of pages, technology available for reproduction of materials (for instance, someone to make slides), technology available to facilitate the presentation (the availability of a slide projector and screen), and format (whether or not to use graphs, whether to have tables in the body of the report or in the appendix). Again, these are best determined before the presentation is organized.

WHAT TO PRESENT AND HOW TO PRESENT IT

To answer the "what" and "how" of presentation, the presenter should gauge the audience and organize the materials in the manner that provides information in a form that is easy to assimilate while still doing justice to the content of the investigation. The remainder of this chapter will focus on the major forms of data presentation and the major questions to be addressed as the findings are interpreted and their implications identified. For the purpose of this chapter, it is assumed that a formal and complete written report of the research endeavor is being made.

The Actual Presentation

Often there is a section of the research report titled "Analysis of Findings." In it the reader expects to find the following topics covered:

1. Description of subjects—demographic or other descriptive physical/biological data,
2. Description of the scores of the subjects on the measures used for independent and dependent variables (and control variables),
3. Findings with respect to the research questions or hypotheses and other findings such as peripheral findings not covered by the research questions that are incidental to the conduct of the study.

Usually, it is best to begin the presentation of findings, especially if it constitutes a separate chapter of the report, with a couple of sentences describing the nature of the study (e.g., descriptive, experimental, correlational, exploratory, etc.), the subjects (e.g., 10-year-old boys, decubitus ulcers, BSN nurses), and the concern being addressed. This serves to refocus the reader on the topic at hand and provides orientation for a reader who elects to read only this section of the report. Less necessary, but often useful as an orientation to the reader, is a topical outline for the presentation of findings. For example, "in this section the research hypotheses will form the structure under which the findings will be presented."

It is helpful to use the list of suggested topics (see paragraph 1 of this section) as an outline for the presentation of suggested findings. If the data lend themselves to the construction of tables and graphs, the task of presenting findings will require little writing. The reader is referred to a particular graph or table for detail by sentences in the narrative that summarize the major inference to be made from the graph or table. An illustration of this is a sentence such as "While the ages of the subjects in the experimental group did not differ from those in the control group, there were proportionately fewer whites and Protestants in the experimental than in the control group (see Table ———)." In this way, the reader can get the gist of the data in the table and is saved from the confusion that may arise as he or she seeks to make sense of many numbers strung out in a narrative that are more comprehensible in a table or graph.

It is appropriate to conclude the presentation of findings with a one-paragraph summary. Even though it may seem redundant, the summary should include a sentence describing the procedure of the study and then sentences giving a *content* summary of the findings with respect to each hypothesis or study question. For example, an adequate summary might be "This retrospective review of the records of 100 adolescents attending the VD clinic indicates that those with high scores on X measure are more likely to do Y; these results were statistically significant. No statistically significant relationships were found between X measure and Z_1 and Z_2."

It is important for the student—and all presenters—to realize that a content summary states fact. A factual statement is one such as "Hypothesis I, that there would be no difference in anxiety before surgery between the group shown the slide-tape presentation about induction of anesthesia and the group shown a slide-tape presentation on the healing process, was rejected." To be avoided are statements such as "In this section the study findings were presented in tables and summarized in the narrative." "Hypothesis I was rejected; the chi-square test indicated a $P > .05$ with 3 degrees of freedom." While this sentence contains information about the statistical test not seen in the content summary, its reference to the hypothesis without indicating the content of the hypothesis places a burden upon the reader to recall the content of Hypothesis I. The statistical procedure employed is a detail that is usually not important enough to be included in the summary.

The next three sections of this chapter discuss the construction and use of tables, graphs, and diagrams in the presentation of findings, followed by a discussion of their interpretation.

TABLES

Tables are useful both for discovering the findings and for presenting them. It is appropriate and expected that tables will be made when there are data describing units consisting of numbers: counts of events or persons with certain attributes or characteristics, scores on tests, numbers measuring phenomena such as weight or blood pressure. Tables may describe units with respect to one variable, such as sex, or many, such as sex, age, and race. Good tables are both technically precise and visually satisfying.

Constructing Tables

The technical aspect of table construction is best approached through an example, in this case the reporting of pupil absence in an elementary school by grade. The data include numbers of days absent for each child in the school and the grade to which each child is assigned. The skeleton outline for the table reporting these data is shown in Figure 14-1. It is customary, but not necessary, to arrange the table so that the independent variable, or the variable by which the units, subjects, or elements are being classified, constitutes the *row* of the table. The dependent variable is placed so that its categories are the *column* headings. The intersections of rows and columns make *cells* into which the raw data are placed. Each object/subject is described by both the independent and dependent variables and thus is counted as a case in a particular cell.

In order to present data in tabular form, it is usually necessary to group the units being described. This grouping may be in terms of categories or in terms of ranges of values with respect to a variable. In the absences from the classroom example, the data are grouped by the

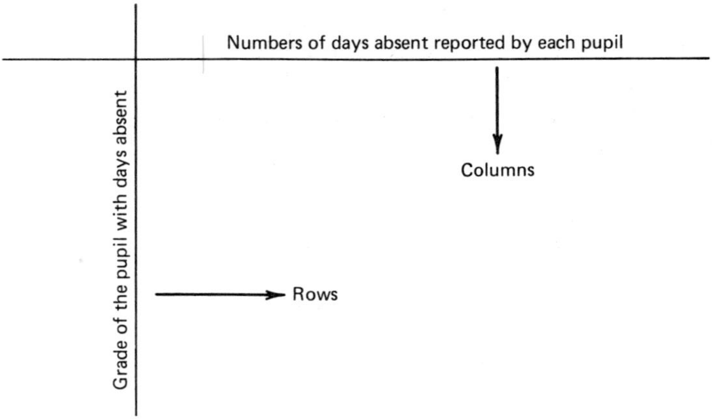

Figure 14-1. Skeleton for a hypothetical table.

child's grade level, and that has been used as the classification scheme for one variable. However, the data have not been grouped for the numbers of days absent. What should be done? It is best to begin the process of establishing groups by discovering the various possible values or characteristics that constitute the measures or categories of the variable, and then to group the data according to the various rules as follows:

- Try to make meaningful categories.
- Try to have the categories cover ranges of values, if not literally, at least practically.
- Try to limit the number of categories so that the table will fit neatly on one page—avoid too many categories.
- If the statistical analysis has already been conducted, the categories should reflect those used for the statistical tests, as appropriate.
- When using numerical data, do not make the intervals greater in range than differences. These differences cannot be ignored.
- If in doubt about the interval, choose the narrower one; intervals can always be combined, but making them smaller requires complete regrouping of the data.
- Uneven intervals can be used, but be sure there is a valid rationale for this.
- At either end of a range of values it is possible to use open categories or intervals.

Thus, in our example, it might be meaningful to group the data into intervals of five days, which comprise a week. But that yields 167 ÷ 5 = 33—too many categories. In that instance it is appropriate to examine the data to determine the frequency with which days absent per pupil fit into each category. A histogram might present these data clearly and leave the table free for the summary. (The construction of histograms is presented in the next section.) If inspection of the data shows higher frequencies at the lower end of the range, the decision might be made to make the following intervals the categories of the dependent variable: 0 days; 1–5 days; 6–10 days; 11–20 days; 21–40 days; more than 40 days.

Once the table has been designed and constructed, it should be given a title. The title should describe the content of the table precisely. Usually, an adequate description of the content of the table evolves if the table is titled in terms of the axes of classification (the row and column headings). This process will be illustrated using our example.

Begin the title with the dependent variable: *Days of Absence During 1978–79.* Then indicate the objects/subjects to whom this refers: *of Pupils.* Next give the independent variable, ways in which the subjects have been classified: *in Grades 1–5* (Fig. 14-2 for an illustration of this). It is possible to give the table a title on the basis of the skeleton. Some researchers think in terms of table titles; then the title can determine the layout of the table. It may be easier for beginners to design the tables—the computer may already have laid them out or they may have evolved during hand tabulation—and then give them titles.

There are several other conventions that should be observed so that each table can stand on its own. Most essential is the title, created in the manner described above. There should be totals both for rows and for columns. This allows the reader to have a ready understanding of the size of each group without having to add the numbers in each cell. This may facilitate on-the-spot calculations of percentages for those who think in such terms. If statistical tests have been done on the data, these should be presented below the table; for example, $\chi^2 = 3.15$, $df = 6$, $ns\alpha = .05$, or $P > .10$ would constitute complete presentation of such data.

The rule about row and column totals presents a problem if the table contains percentages. The rows or columns may not add to 100 as they should because of the rounding that has occurred in each calculation. It is appropriate to present the exact sum, such as 99.8, so that the reader may judge the extent of the errors due to rounding. In other instances, the percentages will not add to 100 because it is possible for an object/subject to have fallen into more than one of the categories of the independent or dependent variables (variables of classification). In this instance the total column should indicate the number of cases that constituted the denominator for the calculation of the percentage; an appropriate label for this row or column would be "total cases" or "total pupils." It is necessary for clarity to present a totals row or column when the data within the table consist of percentages.

Tables can describe objects/subjects in one, two, three, or many more ways. Thus, tables can be said to provide one-way, two-way, and so forth, classifications of the data. The more axes of classification there are, the more difficult it is to organize and present the table. The problem of organization is solved when each variable is considered in terms of whether it is the independent or dependent variable and in terms of its relative importance to the question at hand. In the example above, if the sex of the pupils were known and one wanted to know if boys had a different pattern of absence than girls and if there might be a different pattern by sex and by grade, what arrangement of these data would be most clear? Figure 14-2 shows tables presenting three combinations of variables. These layouts are not the only possibilities, but their presentation indicates how difficult it is to prescribe a format and how much the decision on format can be a matter of fashion or individual preference.

Finally, a word about the visual qualities of the table. Tables should present clear uncluttered views of the findings and analysis. Attention should be paid to the layout of the table: use plenty of space; do not cramp the data. If typing, double space between rows, if possible. Make clear use of upper and lower case letters. For example, presenting the title in upper case letters may set it off nicely from the body of the table. Make judicious use of lines; it is not necessary to construct boxes for each cell of the table—spacing may make the cells quite distinguishable. On the other hand, setting off the axes of classification or totals with lines may contribute to clarity. See Figure 14-3 for an illustration of this.

Deciding When and Where to Present Tables

Tables should be presented to summarize each major finding of the study. Often tables are presented in the text or on separate interleafed pages that follow immediately the page on which reference is made to them. On other occasions such major tables are relegated to the end of a paper; in this case the text should refer the reader to the table by both table number and the page on which it is located.

Layout I: Days Absent from School by Grade and Sex of Pupil

Grade	Sex	*Days Absent* 0	1–5	6–10	etc.	Total
1		0	2	4		
	M	0	2	3		
	F	0	0	1		
2		0	5	10		
	M	0	1	4		
	F	0	4	6		
etc.						
Total						

Layout II: Days Absent from School by Sex and Grade of Pupil

Sex and Grade		*Days Absent* 0	1–5	6–10	etc.	Total
Boys		0	3	7		
	1	0	2	3		
	2	0	1	4		
	etc.					
Girls		0	4	7		
	1	0	0	1		
	2	0	4	6		
	etc.					
Total						

Layout III: Days Absent from School by Sex and Grade of Pupil

	Days Absent 0		1–5		6–10			
Grade	Boys	Girls	Boys	Girls	Boys	Girls	etc.	Total
1	0	0	2	0	3	1		
2	0	0	1	4	4	6		
etc.								
Total								

Figure 14-2. Three layouts for the same data set.

Neat:

TABLE I
DAYS ABSENT FROM SCHOOL BY GRADE PUPIL

	Days Absent						
Grade	*0*	*1–5*	*6–10*	*11–20*	*21–40*	*More than 40*	*Total*
1							
2							
3							
4							
5							
Total							

TABLE I

Not neat: **Days absent From School by Grade pupil**

grade	**0**	**1–5**	**6–10**	**11–20**	**21–40**	**More than 40**	**Total**
1							
2							
3							
4							
5							
TOTAL							

Figure 14-3. Tables Presenting the Same Data: One Neat and One Not Neat

When the sample for the study is small and the variables few in number, a table presenting all data on each case is appropriate. Such a table would be placed in the appendix. If there are too many data for one neat table, the data can be separated. For example, the sociodemographic data may be presented in one table and the data on the other variables in another table.

If it appears that there are too many tables, it may be that tables with only one classification have been constructed and one table summarizing the cases with respect to several variables simultaneously would be more appropriate. A classic, but simplistic, example of this is separate tables to describe the distribution of the sample by race, sex, and age. These data could be more meaningful in one table. Thus, it would be possible for the reader to know if all older persons were black males or white females.

There are instances when reports contain too few tables. This can occur when a correlational analysis is performed, using a statistic such as Pearson's *r,* for example. There is no way that the analysis can be described in tabular form, since continuous data are used. However, it is possible to present the data in a table with the continuous data collapsed into categories. This allows the reader some visual display of the way in which the variables are interrelated. A more appropriate way of visually displaying correlational data is in a graph scattergram, but these are cumbersome to create if the size of the sample exceeds 50 or when multiple correlation is to be portrayed.

Tables represent the ultimate organization of quantitative data. It is well worth the effort to learn to think systematically about the purpose of the study, the relevant data, and how these can be presented. The detail on developing tables in Wandelt (1970, pp. 261–277) will be helpful to the interested student.

GRAPHS

A graph depicts the relation of one variable to another; it represents the variation of one variable or of one or more variables in comparison to another. Graphs are pictorial representations that are constructed by allocating space within an area to the values or descriptors assigned to variables. They convey much information economically.

The simplest graph depicts the frequency with which a certain value or variable occurs in a sample. For example, the weights of student nurses in the entering class have been recorded; the task is to represent this information in a graph. Here, as in the previous example of tables, it is necessary to group the data. The same rules presented earlier for grouping are followed in this instance. As with tables, the graph should have a descriptive title.

If one is constructing a bar graph of the weight data, it might look like that shown in Figure 14-4. Such a bar graph is known as a histogram. When the data being depicted are continuous, it is customary to have each bar abut on the ones adjacent. This makes it easy to visualize the bars of histograms as denoting proportional areas of the total area contained within the histogram. When continuous data are represented as a histogram and the data have been grouped, the extent of variation within categories is not apparent but the distribution of the phenomenon in the sample is indicated. From a bar graph it is not possible to perform statistical computations. However, one can determine the range in which the median falls.

Histograms may be constructed in which the variable being measured

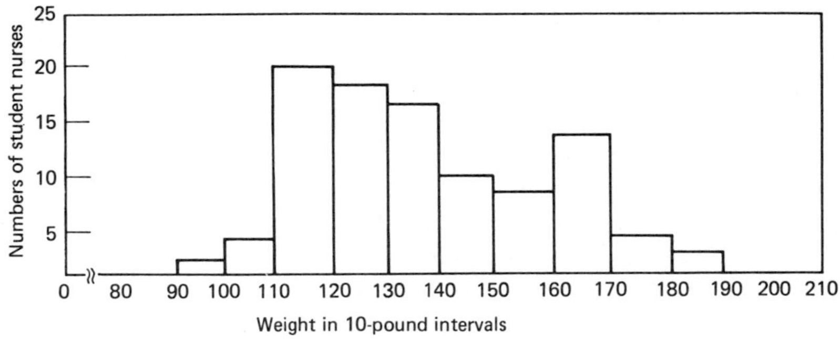

Figure 14-4. Weights of students entering nursing school. ($N = 98$).

is plotted either on the horizontal (*X* axis) or the vertical (*Y* axis) but more commonly in the fashion shown in the example. In order that the reader not be misled, it is important that the intervals on each axis be equal; the interval may be 10 on one axis and 5 on the other, but it must be consistent on each.

More than one variable may be depicted in a bar graph, in which case it is not a histogram. For example, if trends in referrals for follow-up upon hospital discharge over three years are being compared, a graph to convey the numbers of referrals to various agencies could look like Figure 14-5.

Here it is important to note some details of design. The code—either colors or graphics— used for the different entities should be distinct, selected and ordered so that there is a pleasing contrast among them. A key is presented with each code in the order in which it is presented in the graph. The designer may or may not have a rationale for the ordering of the phenomena, but once an order is decided it should be maintained. Do not reorder according to frequency or any other concern once an order is established. A ruler and graph paper may be helpful for making a neat and accurate graph. If the values on an axis do not include zero, it is customary to label the intersection of the *X* and *Y* axis as zero; then place a slash mark through the interval between zero and the lowest number of the range to indicate that it is not to scale or not a possible value.

Bar graphs are particularly useful in oral presentations in which one wishes to be sure the audience understands the message being conveyed. Use of color and design features can add interest to a presentation. However, do not present a histogram to repeat data already conveyed in a table. Generally, use one method or the other for the same data. If it is necessary to convey precise frequencies or percentages, a table may be the mode of choice to present the data. Histograms and tables can be used in the same report. The stem and leaf (Chapter 12) is another graphic form that makes it easy to inspect the data.

DIAGRAMS

Several forms of diagrams are useful in the presentation of data. Diagrams, like tables and graphs, are clear, simple ways to present complex ideas or relationships. Diagrams, like graphs, are helpful when a visual message is thought to be more appropriate than a straight verbal/numerical presentation. None of these is ever presented without accompanying narrative, however.

The *pie diagram* is especially useful when it is necessary to present the

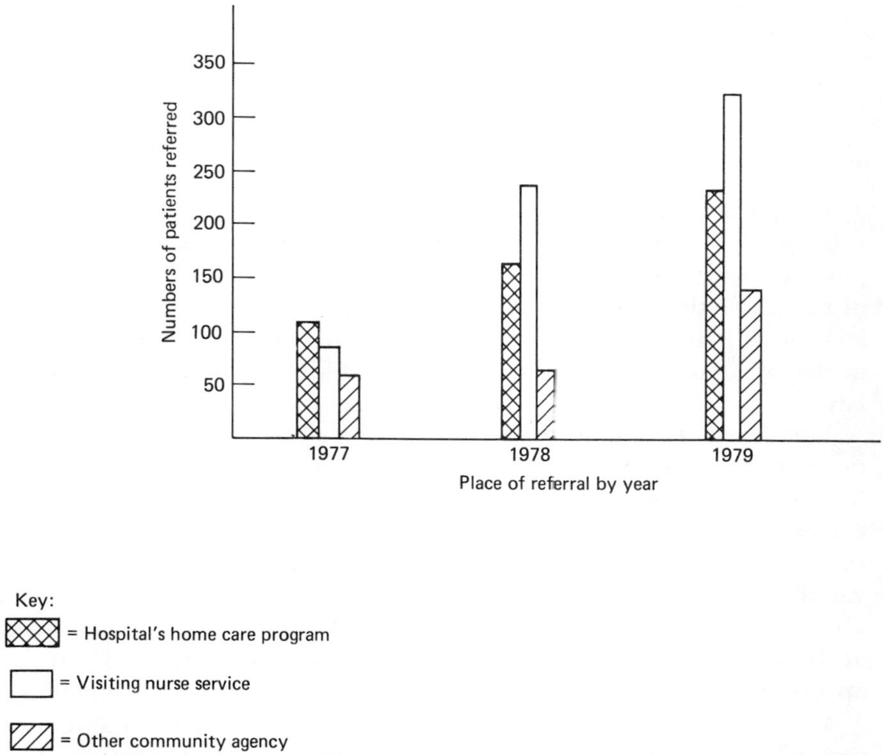

Figure 14-5. Referrals to community agencies from a hospital, 1977–1979.

way in which a particular whole is divided into parts. These diagrams are often used when expenditures of money or effort are being described. Or they may be used to describe the relative contributions of various elements to a whole. For example, a pie diagram can be used to indicate the extent to which various elements are to be represented in the daily caloric intake of a person.

The pie diagram is constructed by conceptualizing the circumference (360°) as equaling 100%. Then, percentages are calculated for each element with the value of the whole (dollars, hours, calories, other units) as the denominator. A protractor is used to divide the circumference according to the number of degrees that correspond to the X% that an element is of the whole. As an illustration, suppose a nurse's 8-hour workday is consumed by patient care (4 hours), conference (3 hours), lunch and break (1 hour). To construct a pie diagram depicting these facts, one first converts the elements into percentages and then calculates the corresponding degrees of the circumference to form the "slice of the pie." These figures are given in the table below:

Element	*Hours*	*Percent of Hours*	
Patient care	4	4 ÷ 8 × 100 = 50%	.50 × 360° = 180°
Conference	3	3 ÷ 8 × 100 = 37.5%	.375 × 360° = 135°
Lunch	1	1 ÷ 8 × 100 = 12.5%	.125 × 360° = 45°

The pie diagram should look like that in Figure 14-6.

Graphics are important. If there are many elements, it may not be possible to write into the segment the label for each one or the percent of the whole that it represents. In such a case, it is necessary to include a key identifying the elements of the diagram. The guidelines discussed in the previous section on bar graphs should be used in developing a key.

A *line diagram* is used when the mathematical relationship between two variables is to be described. For this, one constructs intersecting X (abscissa) and Y (ordinal) axes, marking along each the intervals that correspond to the range of values appropriate to each variable. Usually the independent variable is placed on the Y axis and the dependent variable upon the X axis. An example is given in Figure 14-7. Entries are made by locating the value represented by each case; a dot is placed at the intersection of lines drawn perpendicular to each axis from the appropriate values for each variable. These dots are then connected.

A line diagram also may be used to convey the relative frequencies with which levels of a variable occur. In this instance it is similar to a histogram and is called a frequency polygon, as was presented in

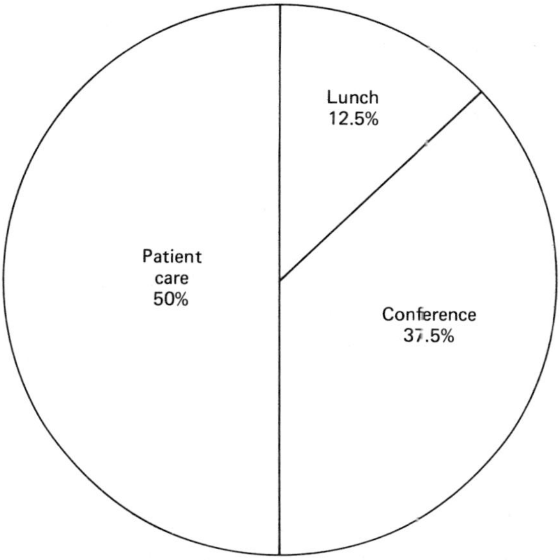

Figure 14-6. Percentage of a nurse's time spent in various activities during an eight hour working day.

Chapter 12. The *X* axis represents levels of intervals of a variable and the *Y* axis the absolute or proportional frequency.

Another use of the line diagram is in the presentation of cumulative frequencies. In this instance the numbers of cases are placed on the *X* axis and the cumulative percentage is placed on the *Y* axis. This form of diagram is useful for determining the number of cases below or above a certain value.

For all of these line diagrams, the convention (discussed in the "Graphs" section) with respect to the slashed line between zero and the first actual interval should be followed.

INTERPRETING THE FINDINGS

The interpretation of findings affords the researcher first voice in critiquing the study design and procedures. In addition, the researcher has the first opportunity to relate the findings to those of others. The interpretation can accord the researcher an opportunity to demonstrate honesty, creativity, and breadth of knowledge with respect to the phenomena under investigation and the methods used in the study of

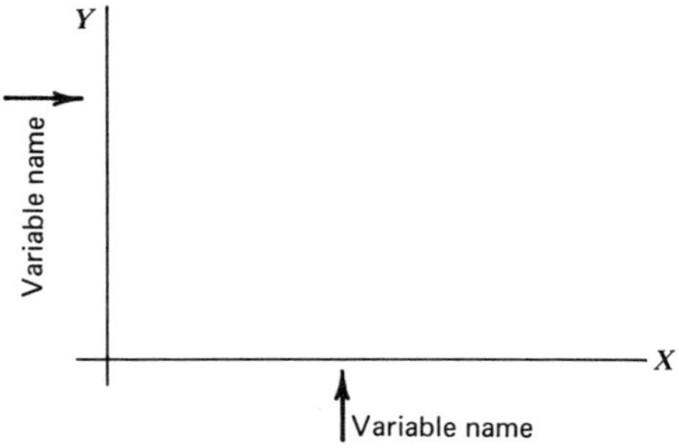

Figure 14-7. Skeleton for a line diagram depicting mathematical relationships. (The *X* and *Y* axes are not included as part of the variable names.)

the phenomena. The interpretation points the way to further work in the area.

Once the data have been analyzed sense must be made of the findings; this step in the research process is called interpretation. Interpretation of findings involves considering the contexts in which the findings must be placed. One context is the immediate situation from which the findings were derived. The other context is the larger one found in the body of knowledge to which the findings relate.

The consideration of contexts is directed to determining the credence and importance to be attached to the findings. In particular, the object of interpretation is to identify *why* the findings are as they are: Was the methodology appropriate and appropriately applied? Was the theory adequate and confirmed by the study? From both of these considerations come implications for practice, for theory, and for further research. These implications and recommendations are also part of the interpretations of the study results.

Items in Interpretation

The major questions to be addressed in the interpretation are presented below. The thoughtful reader will recognize that some of the issues being raised now at the phase of interpretation are identical to those considered during the planning phases of the study. The planning process of the study involved weighing choices for instruments and sampling and procedures in terms of the extent to which they posed threats to reliability and validity. The questions addressed in the interpretation are, in effect, a reassessment of threats to reliability and validity, some of which may not have been known to exist at the planning phase, or were beyond the control of the researcher. Researchers hope for the best with a research design. If all has gone well, "the best" emerges; rarely is this the case, however. More often, one or two factors emerge in a stronger way than were desired and must be weighed as the data are interpreted. Thus, some of the questions listed below may be considered as double checks on the design and subsequent data set. Other questions can only be addressed once the results are known.

Time, Place, Person

First to be considered are the subjects, the setting, and the timing of the study. Was there anything unique about these that would account for the nature of the findings? For example, did some circumstance limit the availability of certain classes of subjects? Or, do you have reason to believe that only certain types of subjects returned the questionnaire? If so, then perhaps the sample does not reflect what was originally intended. This problem frequently arises when the sample is volunteer or the next N patients on a unit. The setting may limit the claims that can be made about the sample; it is possible that even after careful consideration unique characteristics in setting overpower the best sampling procedure and limit the generalizability of the findings even more than was anticipated. Timing and the occurrence of various events before or during the conduct of the study may throw the results in one direction or another either by biasing the selection of the sample or by biasing the responses or behaviors of the subjects. Examples of such events are changes in unit policy where the study is being conducted or newspaper publicity given to the phenomenon being studied just as data collection begins.

Finally, it is important to consider the question: How legitimate is it to extend the findings of this study of an accessible sample to the target population of interest? How reasonable is it to generalize the findings from this group to others, both similar groups in other settings and dissimilar groups in the same setting or in other settings? In other words, are the subjects representative of the larger group? If so, how so? If not, in what ways not? Why not? Does the setting possess characteristics that make it similar to other settings? If so, which ones? Was the phenomenon of interest similar to other phenomena? Which ones? How so?

Standardization of Procedures

Next to be considered are the procedures of the data collection and analysis phases of the study. For example, was it impossible to obtain the posttest scores for both the experimental and control groups at a comparable time following the event of interest? Could all the subjects be tested? With respect to the data analysis, did the expected variation in the independent or dependent variable arise from the subjects' scores or in the measures of the phenomenon of interest? If the variation was not there, how did this effect the analysis? Were the members in the comparison groups uneven to the extent that they rendered the results of statistical tests suspect? Were the results of statistical analysis affected by too small or too large a sample size?

It is important to establish the compatibility of the study findings with the literature. A check on the study results can be accomplished by comparison of the scores and observations and findings to those of other researchers. Examine the scores on independent and dependent variables, acceptance or rejection of hypotheses, and answers to the study questions. Are they similar? If not, what could explain the differences—the setting, subjects, study, study procedures, analysis techniques?

Significance: Statistical and Clinical

An important issue related to the interpretation of results is that of significance. With respect to the variables studied, is statistical significance congruent with practical significance? Differences may be statistically significant but may not matter much in the real world, that is, they may contain no implications for nursing. Nonsignificant results—in the statistical sense—may reflect potentially important differences that have implications for practice or theory. These should be noted, and recommendations for further study or investigation should be made.

Other Problems in Interpretation

All of these factors should be evaluated and incorporated into the research report under discussion as implications, limitations, or recommendations. Consideration of the methodological and theoretical issues discussed above will force the researcher to consider alternative explanations for the study findings. Because most studies are either applications of a new theoretical perspective to a question that has been investigated previously or an extension into a new population or area of a previously developed theoretical framework, the investigator must examine both the theory and the area to which it was applied in the search for alternative explanations for the study findings. One class of explanation relates to the adequacy of the theory on which the study was based, or the framework from which the hypotheses emanated. Does the theory describe what is actually going on? If not, why not?

Another class of explanation could be differences in subjects, measures, setting, or time from previous studies to the current study. Some of these could be differences selected by the researcher, as when one replicates a study of a variable in a teenage population to see if the same variable occurs with equal frequency in a population of middle-aged adults. Other differences often arise in environmental variables beyond the control of the researcher, as when suddenly a policy is changed so that no longer is a certain class of patients admitted to the unit from which the sample was being taken over time. For a discussion organized by whether or not hypotheses are supported, the reader is urged to refer to Polit and Hungler (1978, pp. 599–602).

It is imperative that the researcher consider alternative explanations for the study findings. This allows rationalization of unexpected results and forces careful scrutiny of expected outcomes to determine whether there are other explanations for the results than the one posited by the theory on which the study was based. If there were a number of peculiarities in the study situation, the investigator would want to be cautious and to caution others about the implications of the findings. If the findings conform with the findings of others, this increases confidence in them. If the findings of others are refuted, or are not confirmed, the researcher should raise questions for further investigation, especially if the researcher has confidence in the design and procedures of the study being reported. A major question, in this last instance, would concern the adequacy of the theory or conceptual framework upon which the study was based.

Once the findings have been examined in this way, the researcher can draw conclusions. The major statement of conclusions should relate to the purpose of the study and indicate the facts that emerge from the analysis. The conclusions should be brief.

Out of the conclusions come implications for practice. Because nursing practice encompasses both direct patient care and the development of resources for patient care through education and administration, all three areas should be addressed if at all possible. Even though there are no firm conclusions from the study, it may be that there are implications for practice.

From the conclusions come recommendations for future research. Here, as in the interpretation, both methodological and theoretical concerns should be addressed. Methodological recommendations may refer to replication, sampling, instrumentation, and personnel to conduct the observations. Theoretical concerns may refer to additional variables to consider in subsequent studies or to conceptual or mathematical measurement issues.

SUMMARY

Aspects of data presentation and data interpretation have been presented in this chapter. Data presentation has been conceived to include both the presentation of the research report and presentation of numerical data. In all instances the research report should include a description of the subjects and their selection for participation in the study, the study procedures, and the comparison of the subjects' responses with their earlier responses or the responses of relevant others. The description of subjects and their responses is often given numerical values or placed in categories of descriptors. The presentation of these data in tables and graphs has been recommended, and procedures to be followed have been presented in detail. Desired attributes of all these communications are simplicity and clarity. The interpretation of findings by the investigator places the study results in a methodological and theoretical context. The interpretation allows the reader or listener to understand the significance of the findings and how they relate to the theory used as a conceptual underpinning of the study.

BIBLIOGRAPHY

Polit, D., & Hungler, B. *Nursing Research: Principles and Methods.* Philadelphia: J.B. Lippincott, 1978.

Wandelt, M. *Guide for the Beginning Researcher.* New York: Appleton-Century-Crofts, 1970.

Ward, M. J., & Fettler, M. E. "Research Q and A: What guidelines should be followed in critically evaluating research reports?" *Nursing Research,* March/April, 1979, *28*, pp. 120–126.

15
Critiquing and Reporting

The process of critiquing and reporting research studies is a vital aspect of the discipline of nursing. That is true for most professional nurses, but it is especially true for those nurses interested in research. Even though this book has presented the information needed to critique a research article and to prepare a review for publication, this chapter integrates that information to assist the student in the use of these materials. The purpose of this chapter is to present the fundamentals of critiquing and to describe a method for reporting research studies for publication in journals. Critiquing is discussed before reporting, because the skills necessary for good critiquing are employed in reporting, especially when publication is intended.

CRITIQUING

Critiquing is the thoughtful examination of a research report and consideration of the sources of the hypotheses, the concept of the study, the appropriateness of the method used, the validity of the conclusions, and the manner of presenting the study. Critiquing is constructive criticism and evaluation. It avoids nit-picking comments and minor details.

Critiquing the research efforts of others is an important aspect of learning methods of conducting research because it helps the critic to develop the ability to identify the strengths and weaknesses in his or her own research studies. The critic learns also to think critically, using all available knowledge. The main purpose of a critique is to assess the strength and weaknesses of a study, a report, or an article. To achieve that purpose requires the objective judgment of the critic. This book has presented the material needed by the student to critique a research article. This section discusses specific aspects of the critiquing process: the advantages, the limitations, and a method for critiquing.

Advantages and Limitations of Critiquing

Reading a critique of a research article has advantages and limitations compared with reading the entire article. It permits the reader to gather information quickly but carries the risk of overlooking something important. In the beginning, the student should read entire articles and good critiques of those same articles. A student learns from such examples the advantages and limitations of condensation and critical comment. In the end, learning to critique is learning by doing and benefiting from the criticisms of faculty members and colleagues. The student needs a fairly thorough knowledge of the subject matter and of research methods before being able to prepare a good critique.

Major limitations many students have in critiquing articles are lack of critical thinking ability and lack of familiarity with the subject matter (Selltiz, Wrightsman, and Cook, 1976). Critical thinking constitutes the application of the universal criteria of logical adequacy and logical consistency. Familiarity with the subject matter refers to knowledge of the natural history of the focus of the study. Students who lack critical thinking ability and familiarity with the subject matter may not be confident in their abilities as critics. Practice and time will overcome most of those limitations. But a valid critique always depends on the knowledge of the critic. Some knowledge of the methods of critiquing will also prove helpful to students.

How to Critique

Critiquing a research article involves identifying answers to questions. This section presents the questions that need to be answered. The outline used for critiquing is the same as the outline used in the development of a research project. It includes the problem, literature review, hypotheses, method, data analysis, findings, and conclusion.

The Problem

In critiquing a research article, the student first considers the statement of the problem examined by the study. What is the objective? Or what is the topic to be explored and why? This statement should give the reasons for undertaking the study. Further, the relevant background information should lead from a general to a specific problem that is viewed as important and feasible to study. The critic would be interested in knowing what, if any, solutions to the specific problem previous research had achieved. General problem statements ask good questions but usually are too broad to be researchable. Therefore, the general problem needs to be subdivided into several specific problems. The critic should be able to recognize whether the statement addresses a practical problem or a theoretical one. Study of these two types of problems is sometimes called *applied research* and *basic research,* respectively. A practical problem may provide more immediately usable answers but a theoretical one may be more important. There is, however, no sharp dividing line between the two types. They usually overlap with elements of both types in most research studies.

The following questions are the most useful ones for critiquing problem statements:

1. What is the problem?
2. Is it clearly stated?
3. Is it important and why?
4. Is it possible to apply research methods to the problem, or, in other words, can the relevant data be obtained?
5. Are the background reasons and conceptual framework understandable?

Literature Review

In critiquing an article, the critic should not consider the literature review the most important step. Unless the student has a thorough knowledge of the available literature, judging its completeness may be difficult. For this reason, the literature review associated with an article must be judged primarily on the basis of the relevance of the review, its aptness, and its cogency. Although the dates of citations give a clue to the time period represented by the literature review, the review should not necessarily be exhaustive and should not contain irrelevant citations. Further, newer citations should not always be favored over older ones. Relevance is the most important consideration.

The literature review should provide some historical perspective and explain the evolution of the statements of the problem and how it relates to the extant body of knowledge. In this way the literature review justifies and explains the hypotheses developed for the study.

Hypotheses

Hypotheses are tentative assumptions that are thought to be true but for which there is no empirical evidence that enables a person to decide whether they are actually true. Another way of defining hypotheses is as formulations of ideas in such a way that their support can be demonstrated by obtaining appropriate and valid empirical evidence. Hypotheses start in the mind of the researcher based on experience and reading the literature (Fox, 1976). Hypotheses rarely emerge in complete form at one time. They grow by thinking and discussion and reading.

It is essential for the critic to identify the hypotheses of the research article he or she is critiquing. Then, the hypotheses should be considered for clarity, relevance to the problem, and the extent to which they deal with the whole problem. It is frequently found that hypotheses are concerned with only a part of the problem. Many problems are too big or too complex to be solved by a single study.

The next step, after identifying the hypotheses, is to consider how the hypotheses are to be tested. What independent variables are to be included and what dependent variables will be measured? Are the variables meaningful and realistic (Abdellah and Levine, 1971)? In addition, the student evaluates the extent of the relationship indicated among the variables (Treece and Treece, 1977). The student asks 1) are the hypotheses testable; 2) are they based on findings of other studies, facts, theories (Abdellah and Levine); 3) are the variables operationally defined (Treece and Treece, 1977); 4) will the identified relationships be causal, associative, or spurious (Abdellah and Levine, 1971); and 5) are the underlying concepts important and do they justify the study (Fleming and Hayden, 1974)? A critique of the hypotheses will lead directly into consideration of the research method described in the article.

Method

As the student knows, the method of a study is the orderly arrangement of its scientific inquiry in a research design. The student approaches the critique of this section with the format used in the preparation of a study. The format includes identifying and defining the variables, choosing among alternative data collection methods, and the sampling frame. In reviewing the variables, the student considers their characteristics, traits, elements, and whether they are independent or dependent. This consideration is especially important in relation to the specific research design, that is, experimental, quasi-experimental, descriptive, or other. Recall that the dependent and independent variables are the cornerstones of experimental studies and would require careful attention. The student notes how the author identified the variables and their roles in the study.

An important aspect of critiquing the method is examining definitions of the variables. Especially important are the indications of the measurement values associated with each of the variables. It is important that measurement values are appropriate to the variables being studied. In addition, the student should examine the operational definitions of the variables and the clarity of instructions for the treatment of the variables.

Another component to critique in the method section of an article is the data collection. Data may have been collected in one or more ways, such as surveys, observations, extracts from medical records, participant observation, interviews, or questionnaires. If questionnaires were used, the student would want to know whether they had been developed by the author, pretested for item construction and inclusion, and also tested for reliability and validity. The student would also note whether or not the questionnaire were included in the article. If an instrument developed by someone else had been used, the student should see whether or not the author listed its origin.

Sampling is the last factor to consider in the critique of the research method. Students should consider the topic, who the subjects are, the procedures used for selecting them, and from what larger population (the universe) they came. To what extent does the sample selection process assure that the sample is representative of the universe? Finally, the student evaluates the adequacy of the sample size and whether attention has been paid to protecting human rights and to obtaining informed consent from subjects who agree to participate in the study.

Data Analysis

Critiquing the data analysis section of a research article would involve the following questions: First, is the presentation of the data clear? Are the tabulations relevant? If the study is a quantitative one, what mathematical manipulations were applied? What statistical tests were used? Were the tests used correctly? What significant conclusions were reached? What interpretation was applied to the conclusions in relation to the hypotheses and purpose of the study (Batey, 1970)? What importance was attached to any nonsignificant findings (Polit and Hungler, 1978)? Negative findings are often as important as positive findings, although not as exciting.

A second aspect of the data analysis review is to consider the nature of the study population, its geographic distribution, and the response rate. Was attention paid to the characteristics of those who did not respond?

The student then evaluates the relationship of the data and its analyses to the hypotheses and to the problem under study. When this aspect of the critique has been completed, the student advances to the findings and the summary of the research article.

Findings

Critiquing the findings of a research article is relatively simple. The student, at this point, has considered the problem, literature review, hypotheses, data collection methods, and data analysis. The findings should be based on and should flow from all of those areas, especially the data. The findings should be presented in such a way that the data almost speak for themselves. The critique considers whether, in fact, the data are clearly displayed.

Conclusion or Summary

The interpretation of the data and findings and statements of statistical validity make up the conclusion, which summarizes in concise language the new information uncovered by the study. The critic judges whether the conclusion is supported by the data.

In summary, critiquing a research article requires that the student evaluate the material presented in relation to the research objective and protocol. The student should be able to recognize the strengths and limitations of the study, especially whether the conclusion is soundly based on the empirical evidence.

REPORT WRITING FOR PUBLICATION

Reporting is the culmination of the research process. At the conclusion of a research study, investigators feel obligated to report the outcomes of the study so that others can benefit from the findings. The reasons underlying the communication would vary depending upon the circumstances of the study. Reporting may be necessary in return for funds provided by foundations or grants (see Abdellah and Levine, 1971, pp. 608–646, for a full presentation of funding sources). Reporting also may be a requirement of an educational program, such as for an advanced degree. Articles written for publication are part of the scholarly exchange of ideas, which stimulate and generate progress in science and technology. Presentation of papers and oral reports at conference is also part of this exchange but is based on written reports. This section discusses methods for preparing a written research report for publication.

Writing an Article for Publication

In considering an article for publication, students in nursing may ask: "Why would I want to publish?" One answer to that question may be that the maintenance of nursing as a professional group depends on nurses sharing their knowledge and achievements with as many other health professionals as possible. Additions to nursing knowledge should become widely known through publication in the professional literature of the health fields (Styles, 1978). To fulfill that objective, nursing students should learn the basic skills and format used in writing an article for publication. There are other reasons. In one classroom, students were required to prepare an article as though for publication in which research outcomes were presented. This was one aspect of a research course offered to nursing students seeking a baccalaureate degree (The Johns Hopkins University Nursing Education Programs, 1977).

Many students feel that writing for publication or writing for any reason is difficult. Writing is never easy. The difficulty, however, can be diminished if students practice writing and follow some constructive suggestions. First, students should prepare an outline for each section. Second, they should begin with the section that is uppermost in mind and write a draft of that section, using the notes that have accumulated during the literature review and the study itself. As ideas are formed, they should be written down in anticipation of writing a report (Barzun and Graff, 1977). After writing each section, students should let it rest for a few days to allow opportunity for further thought. After a reasonable but not excessive time students should reread and rewrite the section. Often errors will be discovered, and awkward, unclear expressions will be found that need polishing. Each section should be treated in this fashion. Students are directed to Bestor (1976, Part II) and Barzun (1976, Part VI) for helpful suggestions on writing revisions.

Some experienced writers suggest that the beginning of the article should be written last. In this way, students may be able to write a more coherent report, logically proceeding from the beginning to a firm conclusion.

In addition to the suggestions presented above, there are pitfalls to be avoided in writing. First, avoid flowery expressions, remembering that the article is a report of facts rather than feelings. Second, use clear grammar with attention to verb tenses. Use the past tense, since the study has already been completed. Finally, beware of redundance, repetition, excessive verbiage, and clumsy wording. Use adverbs sparingly. Avoid not only unnecessary complexity but also excessive compression and qualification (Crichton, 1975). Note the cautions that were presented in Chapter 5 on the use of quotations. Most important, avoid procrastination. The only real way to learn to write is to write, rewrite, and write again.

Format Used for Publication

The successful and clear development of an article for publication often depends on the use of an outline to guide its preparation. The following is a suggested outline that students have found helpful:

1. Introduction. The introduction should include a brief statement of the problem, placing the study purpose in the last sentence. In that way, readers can easily identify the nature of the study, and the article will have established a beginning point for the reader.

2. Literature review. The review may be presented as a separate section or incorporated into the content of the article. Most journals prefer that literature reviews be made a part of the body of an article. This section should include results of prior research and appropriate concepts relating to the study.

3. Hypotheses. Some studies, such as those that are of a descriptive nature, may have no hypotheses. However, if, as in most studies, the student has tested hypotheses, they should be stated clearly. This should be a separate section of the article for emphasis.

4. Method. This section could be divided into subcategories, such as 1) setting, 2) sample selection, 3) data collection, 4) statistical tests, and 5) data analysis. The reader is urged to review Chapter 14 of this book for a presentation of tables and Chapters 12 and 13 for statistical analysis.

5. Findings. Findings should be firmly based on the data and the hypotheses. Speculation should be avoided.

6. Limitations of the study. It is desirable to state what the study was unable to do. The discussion of limitations should include a statement about variables that were not or could not be controlled.

7. Discussion of study findings. This section relates the findings to prior research and prior knowledge and to the hypotheses.

8. Conclusion. The conclusion provides a brief summary of what was found, which hypotheses were supported, and which were not supported. It may include recommendations for further studies.

10. References. These include both published and unpublished materials.

11. Abstract. The abstract consists of a single paragraph summary of the study report without any detail.

If this type of outline is followed, the writer will have presented an article that is clear and understandable. As previously stated, the article must be revised, rewritten as needed, and edited for typographical errors before it is submitted for publication. The specific format requirements of the journal to which the article will be submitted must be followed.

Abstracts deserve special attention. Students may find this to be the most difficult aspect of reporting. An abstract is a summary of the study report, and it can be written only after the study and the report are completed. The length of an abstract should be about 200 words or less and should include the purpose of the study, the type of study, and a statement of the principal findings. The abstract, usually printed between the title and the first paragraph, helps the reader know the nature of the article without having to read the entire article. It should be a brief but "comprehensive summary of the observations and conclusions of the original article" (French, 1968, p. 120). Developing an abstract of a student's study serves several purposes. It provides a student with the opportunity to practice "condensation and selective organization . . ." (Taylor, 1967, p. 62). It also helps a student to gain a succinct understanding of the study.

Steps in Submitting an Article for Publication

When a study has been completed, the student, for either educational or personal reasons, may wish to submit an article for publication. At that time it must be decided where to submit the article. The first step in gaining the answer to that question is to peruse the journals, especially those that publish articles related to the study topic. Some of these journals relate to nursing and are published by nursing organizations. The student knows that nursing journals include, for example, *Nursing Research, American Journal of Nursing, Nursing Outlook, Nursing Forum, Nursing '81, Research in Nursing and Health,* and others for specific clinical areas. However, the student may find that the topic does not fit into any of the nursing journals. In that event other journals that focus on specific topics relevant to health care can be considered. These may include journals such as *Hospitals (JAHA), The American Journal of Public Health,* and *The New England Journal of Medicine.* These and other journals accept articles submitted by nurses. If the student is undecided about the appropriateness of a journal, it would be wise to seek advice from a faculty member, an experienced writer, or a librarian. The student probably will have more than one journal in mind for possible publication of the manuscript.

With one or more journals identified, the student should review the journal's editorial policies. Policy directives are found in each issue of a journal and usually include the journal's preferences for topics, format, style, typical length of articles, number and kind of copies to submit (i.e., an original and a number of duplicate copies), and, perhaps, the expected time lapse for editorial decisions. Before submitting a manuscript, the student should have another person review the manuscript to ensure that it is grammatically correct and that it is clear and understandable. With the manuscript reviewed and a journal identified, the student may write to the editor inquiring about the journal's interest in receiving the article. If that is not desirable, the student mails the manuscript, in the prescribed form, and awaits the editor's response.

Before deciding on acceptance or rejection of a submitted article, the editor of the journal usually has the manuscript reviewed by one or more members of a review board, which usually consists of volunteer experts. After that review, the author will receive notification from the editor indicating the decision. If the article is rejected, the editor's reply will usually include the reasons underlying the decision and may include suggestions for revision. When articles are rejected, the author may or may not be encouraged to submit the manuscript to another appropriate journal. Letters indicating the acceptance of manuscripts will usually include the projected date of publication, which is often many months in the future.

Submitting an article for publication to a referred journal, that is, one with a review board, is a valuable experience. Students, whether going into nursing practice or advanced education, will find the experience worthwhile and should prepare and submit manuscripts for publication. These manuscripts may include review articles of the work of others in addition to reports of original studies or observations.

SUMMARY

This chapter has presented the methods for critiquing and reporting research articles. The student should now realize that understanding the research process is essential to critiquing research reports and published articles of research studies. Further, the student should be aware that critiquing and reporting help the researcher to sharpen his or her analytical skills and to increase knowledge. Critiques and articles are important parts of the exchange of information essential to the research enterprise. The logical organization of material related to problem identification, study purposes, hypotheses, data analysis, findings, summary, and references is a skill acquired through practice. Scholarly thinking is strengthened as students learn the strengths and weaknesses of research studies conducted by others and learn how to prepare research articles for publication.

BIBLIOGRAPHY

Abdellah, F. G., & Levine, E. *Better Patient Care Through Nursing Research.* New York: Macmillan, 1971.

Barzun, J. *Simple and Direct: A Rhetoric for Writers.* New York: Harper & Row, 1976.

Barzun, J., & Graff, H. F. *The Modern Researcher.* 3rd edition. New York: Harcourt Brace Jovanovich, 1977.

Batey, M. V. Methodological issues in research, in *Communicating Nursing Research,* Vol. 3. Boulder, Colorado: WICHE, 1970.

Bestor, D. K. Writing an article for publication: Part two. *Nurse Practitioner,* May/June, 1976, *3,* No. 5, pp. 21–23.

Crichton, M. Medical obfuscation: Structure and function. *New England Journal of Medicine,* December 11, 1975, *293,* No. 24, pp. 1257–1259.

Fleming, J. W., & Hayden, J. Reading research reports critically. *Nursing Outlook,* March, 1974, *22,* No. 3, pp. 172–175.

Fox, D. J. *Fundamentals of Research in Nursing,* 3rd edition. New York: Appleton-Century-Crofts, 1976, p. 288.

French, R. M. *The Dynamics of Health Care,* 2nd edition. New York: McGraw-Hill, 1974.

Polit, D. F., & Hungler, B. P. *Nursing Research: Principles and Methods.* Philadelphia: J.B. Lippincott, 1978.

Selltiz, C., Wrightsman, L. S., & Cook, S. W. *Research Methods in Social Relations,* 3rd edition. New York: Holt, Rinehart & Winston, 1976.

Styles, M. M. Why publish? *Image,* June, 1978, *10,* No. 2, pp. 28–31.

Taylor, S. D. How to prepare an abstract. *Nursing Outlook,* September, 1967, *15,* No. 9, pp. 61–63.

Treece, E. W., & Treece, J. W. *Elements of Research in Nursing,* 2nd edition. St. Louis: C. V. Mosby, 1977.

Appendices: Selected Statistical Tables

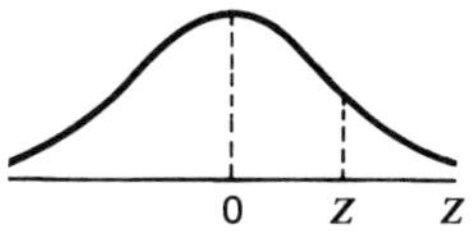

Table A. Cumulative Normal Frequency Distribution
(Area Under the Standard Normal Curve from 0 to Z)

Z	*0.00*	*0.01*	*0.02*	*0.03*	*0.04*	*0.05*	*0.06*	*0.07*	*0.08*	*0.09*
0.0	0.0000	0.0040	0.0080	0.0120	0.0160	0.0199	0.0239	0.0279	0.0319	0.0359
0.1	.0398	.0438	.0478	.0517	.0557	.0596	.0636	.0675	.0714	.0753
0.2	.0793	.0832	.0871	.0910	.0948	.0987	.1026	.1064	.1103	.1141
0.3	.1179	.1217	.1255	.1293	.1331	.1368	.1406	.1443	.1480	.1517
0.4	.1554	.1591	.1628	.1664	.1700	.1736	.1772	.1808	.1844	.1879
0.5	.1915	.1950	.1985	.2019	.2054	.2088	.2123	.2157	.2190	.2224
0.6	.2257	.2291	.2324	.2357	.2389	.2422	.2454	.2486	.2517	.2549
0.7	.2580	.2611	.2642	.2673	.2704	.2734	.2764	.2794	.2823	.2852
0.8	.2881	.2910	.2939	.2967	.2995	.3023	.3051	.3078	.3106	.3133
0.9	.3159	.3186	.3212	.3238	.3264	.3289	.3315	.3340	.3365	.3389
1.0	.3413	.3438	.3461	.3485	.3508	.3531	.3554	.3577	.3599	.3621
1.1	.3643	.3665	.3686	.3708	.3729	.3749	.3770	.3790	.3810	.3830
1.2	.3849	.3869	.3888	.3907	.3925	.3944	.3962	.3980	.3997	.4015
1.3	.4032	.4049	.4066	.4082	.4099	.4115	.4131	.4147	.4162	.4177
1.4	.4192	.4207	.4222	.4236	.4251	.4265	.4279	.4292	.4306	.4319

1.5	.4332	.4345	.4357	.4370	.4382	.4394	.4406	.4418	.4429	.4441
1.6	.4452	.4463	.4474	.4484	.4495	.4505	.4515	.4525	.4535	.4545
1.7	.4554	.4564	.4573	.4582	.4591	.4599	.4608	.4616	.4625	.4633
1.8	.4641	.4649	.4656	.4664	.4671	.4678	.4686	.4693	.4699	.4706
1.9	.4713	.4719	.4726	.4732	.4738	.4744	.4750	.4756	.4761	.4767
2.0	.4772	.4778	.4783	.4788	.4793	.4798	.4803	.4808	.4812	.4817
2.1	.4821	.4826	.4830	.4834	.4838	.4842	.4846	.4850	.4854	.4857
2.2	.4861	.4864	.4868	.4871	.4875	.4878	.4881	.4884	.4887	.4890
2.3	.4893	.4896	.4898	.4901	.4904	.4906	.4909	.4911	.4913	.4916
2.4	.4918	.4920	.4922	.4925	.4927	.4929	.4931	.4932	.4934	.4936
2.5	.4938	.4940	.4941	.4943	.4945	.4946	.4948	.4949	.4951	.4952
2.6	.4953	.4955	.4956	.4957	.4959	.4960	.4961	.4962	.4963	.4964
2.7	.4965	.4966	.4967	.4968	.4969	.4970	.4971	.4972	.4973	.4974
2.8	.4974	.4975	.4976	.4977	.4977	.4978	.4979	.4979	.4980	.4981
2.9	.4981	.4982	.4982	.4983	.4984	.4984	.4985	.4985	.4986	.4986
3.0	.4987	.4987	.4987	.4988	.4988	.4989	.4989	.4989	.4990	.4990
3.1	.4990	.4991	.4991	.4991	.4992	.4992	.4992	.4992	.4993	.4993
3.2	.4993	.4993	.4994	.4994	.4994	.4994	.4994	.4995	.4995	.4995
3.3	.4995	.4995	.4995	.4996	.4996	.4996	.4996	.4996	.4996	.4997
3.4	.4997	.4997	.4997	.4997	.4997	.4997	.4997	.4997	.4997	.4998
3.6	.4998	.4998	.4999	.4999	.4999	.4999	.4999	.4999	.4999	.4999
3.9	.5000									

SOURCE: Reprinted by permission from *Statistical Methods* by George W. Snedecor & William G. Cochran, Sixth Edition, © 1967 by The Iowa State University Press, Ames, Iowa.

Table B. The t Distribution

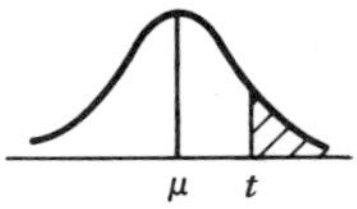

df	$t_{.10}$	$t_{.05}$	$t_{.025}$	$t_{.01}$	$t_{.005}$
1	3.078	6.3138	12.706	31.821	63.657
2	1.886	2.9200	4.3027	6.965	9.9248
3	1.638	2.3534	3.1825	4.541	5.8409
4	1.533	2.1318	2.7764	3.747	4.6041
5	1.476	2.0150	2.5706	3.365	4.0321
6	1.440	1.9432	2.4469	3.143	3.7074
7	1.415	1.8946	2.3646	2.998	3.4995
8	1.397	1.8595	2.3060	2.896	3.3554
9	1.383	1.8331	2.2622	2.821	3.2498
10	1.372	1.8125	2.2281	2.764	3.1693
11	1.363	1.7959	2.2010	2.718	3.1058
12	1.356	1.7823	2.1788	2.681	3.0545
13	1.350	1.7709	2.1604	2.650	3.0123
14	1.345	1.7613	2.1448	2.624	2.9768
15	1.341	1.7530	2.1315	2.602	2.9467
16	1.337	1.7459	2.1199	2.583	2.9208
17	1.333	1.7396	2.1098	2.567	2.8982
18	1.330	1.7341	2.1009	2.552	2.8784
19	1.328	1.7291	2.0930	2.539	2.8609
20	1.325	1.7247	2.0860	2.528	2.8453
21	1.323	1.7207	2.0796	2.518	2.8314
22	1.321	1.7171	2.0739	2.508	2.8188
23	1.319	1.7139	2.0687	2.500	2.8073
24	1.318	1.7109	2.0639	2.492	2.7969
25	1.316	1.7081	2.0595	2.485	2.7874
26	1.315	1.7056	2.0555	2.479	2.7787
27	1.314	1.7033	2.0518	2.473	2.7707

Table B. *(Continued)*

df	$t_{.10}$	$t_{.05}$	$t_{.025}$	$t_{.01}$	$t_{.005}$
28	1.313	1.7011	2.0484	2.467	2.7633
29	1.311	1.6991	2.0452	2.462	2.7564
30	1.310	1.6973	2.0423	2.457	2.7500
35	1.3062	1.6896	2.0301	2.438	2.7239
40	1.3031	1.6839	2.0211	2.423	2.7045
45	1.3007	1.6794	2.0141	2.412	2.6896
50	1.2987	1.6759	2.0086	2.403	2.6778
60	1.2959	1.6707	2.0003	2.390	2.6603
70	1.2938	1.6669	1.9945	2.381	2.6480
80	1.2922	1.6641	1.9901	2.374	2.6388
90	1.2910	1.6620	1.9867	2.368	2.6316
100	1.2901	1.6602	1.9840	2.364	2.6260
120	1.2887	1.6577	1.9799	2.358	2.6175
140	1.2876	1.6558	1.9771	2.353	2.6114
160	1.2869	1.6545	1.9749	2.350	2.6070
180	1.2863	1.6534	1.9733	2.347	2.6035
200	1.2858	1.6525	1.9719	2.345	2.6006
∞	1.282	1.645	1.96	2.326	2.576

SOURCE: CIBA-Geigy, *Documenta Geigy, Scientific Tables*, 7th ed., 1970. Reproduced with permission of CIBA-Geigy Corp.

Table C. Critical Values of Spearman's Rank Correlation Coefficient

$\alpha(2)$:	0.50	0.20	0.10	0.05	0.02	0.01	0.005	0.002	0.001
$\alpha(1)$:	0.25	0.10	0.05	0.025	0.01	0.005	0.0025	0.001	0.0005
n									
4	0.600	1.000	1.000						
5	0.500	0.800	0.900	1.000	1.000				
6	0.371	0.657	0.829	0.886	0.943	1.000	1.000		
7	0.321	0.571	0.714	0.786	0.893	0.929	0.964	1.000	1.000
8	0.310	0.524	0.643	0.738	0.833	0.881	0.905	0.952	0.976
9	0.267	0.483	0.600	0.700	0.783	0.833	0.867	0.917	0.933
10	0.248	0.455	0.564	0.648	0.745	0.794	0.830	0.879	0.903
11	0.236	0.427	0.536	0.618	0.709	0.755	0.800	0.845	0.873
12	0.217	0.406	0.503	0.587	0.678	0.727	0.769	0.818	0.846
13	0.209	0.385	0.484	0.560	0.648	0.703	0.747	0.791	0.824
14	0.200	0.367	0.464	0.538	0.626	0.679	0.723	0.771	0.802
15	0.189	0.354	0.446	0.521	0.604	0.654	0.700	0.750	0.779
16	0.182	0.341	0.429	0.503	0.582	0.635	0.679	0.729	0.762
17	0.176	0.328	0.414	0.485	0.566	0.615	0.662	0.713	0.748
18	0.170	0.317	0.401	0.472	0.550	0.600	0.643	0.695	0.728
19	0.165	0.309	0.391	0.460	0.535	0.584	0.628	0.677	0.712
20	0.161	0.299	0.380	0.447	0.520	0.570	0.612	0.662	0.696
21	0.156	0.292	0.370	0.435	0.508	0.556	0.599	0.648	0.681
22	0.152	0.284	0.361	0.425	0.496	0.544	0.586	0.634	0.667
23	0.148	0.278	0.353	0.415	0.486	0.532	0.573	0.622	0.654
24	0.144	0.271	0.344	0.406	0.476	0.521	0.562	0.610	0.642
25	0.142	0.265	0.337	0.398	0.466	0.511	0.551	0.598	0.630

26	0.138	0.259	0.331	0.390	0.457	0.501	0.541	0.587	0.619
27	0.136	0.255	0.324	0.382	0.448	0.491	0.531	0.577	0.608
28	0.133	0.250	0.317	0.375	0.440	0.483	0.522	0.567	0.598
29	0.130	0.245	0.312	0.368	0.433	0.475	0.513	0.558	0.589
30	0.128	0.240	0.306	0.362	0.425	0.467	0.504	0.549	0.580
31	0.126	0.236	0.301	0.356	0.418	0.459	0.496	0.541	0.571
32	0.124	0.232	0.296	0.350	0.412	0.452	0.489	0.533	0.563
33	0.121	0.229	0.291	0.345	0.405	0.446	0.482	0.525	0.554
34	0.120	0.225	0.287	0.340	0.399	0.439	0.475	0.517	0.547
35	0.118	0.222	0.283	0.335	0.394	0.433	0.468	0.510	0.539
36	0.116	0.219	0.279	0.330	0.388	0.427	0.462	0.504	0.533
37	0.114	0.216	0.275	0.325	0.383	0.421	0.456	0.497	0.526
38	0.113	0.212	0.271	0.321	0.378	0.415	0.450	0.491	0.519
39	0.111	0.210	0.267	0.317	0.373	0.410	0.444	0.485	0.513
40	0.110	0.207	0.264	0.313	0.368	0.405	0.439	0.479	0.507
41	0.108	0.204	0.261	0.309	0.364	0.400	0.433	0.473	0.501
42	0.107	0.202	0.257	0.305	0.359	0.395	0.428	0.468	0.495
43	0.105	0.199	0.254	0.301	0.355	0.391	0.423	0.463	0.490
44	0.104	0.197	0.251	0.298	0.351	0.386	0.419	0.458	0.484
45	0.103	0.194	0.248	0.294	0.347	0.382	0.414	0.453	0.479
46	0.102	0.192	0.246	0.291	0.343	0.378	0.410	0.448	0.474
47	0.101	0.190	0.243	0.288	0.340	0.374	0.405	0.443	0.469
48	0.100	0.188	0.240	0.285	0.336	0.370	0.401	0.439	0.465
49	0.098	0.186	0.238	0.282	0.333	0.366	0.397	0.434	0.460
50	0.097	0.184	0.235	0.279	0.329	0.363	0.393	0.430	0.456

Table C. *(Continued)*

$\alpha(2)$:	0.50	0.20	0.10	0.05	0.02	0.01	0.005	0.002	0.001
$\alpha(1)$:	0.25	0.10	0.05	0.025	0.01	0.005	0.0025	0.001	0.0005
n									
51	0.096	0.182	0.233	0.276	0.326	0.359	0.390	0.426	0.451
52	0.095	0.180	0.231	0.274	0.323	0.356	0.386	0.422	0.447
53	0.095	0.179	0.228	0.271	0.320	0.352	0.382	0.418	0.443
54	0.094	0.177	0.226	0.268	0.317	0.349	0.379	0.414	0.439
55	0.093	0.175	0.224	0.266	0.314	0.346	0.375	0.411	0.435
56	0.092	0.174	0.222	0.264	0.311	0.343	0.372	0.407	0.432
57	0.091	0.172	0.220	0.261	0.308	0.340	0.369	0.404	0.428
58	0.090	0.171	0.218	0.259	0.306	0.337	0.366	0.400	0.424
59	0.089	0.169	0.216	0.257	0.303	0.334	0.363	0.397	0.421
60	0.089	0.168	0.214	0.255	0.300	0.331	0.360	0.394	0.418
61	0.088	0.166	0.213	0.252	0.298	0.329	0.357	0.391	0.414
62	0.087	0.165	0.211	0.250	0.296	0.326	0.354	0.388	0.411
63	0.086	0.163	0.209	0.248	0.293	0.323	0.351	0.385	0.408
64	0.086	0.162	0.207	0.246	0.291	0.321	0.348	0.382	0.405
65	0.085	0.161	0.206	0.244	0.289	0.318	0.346	0.379	0.402
66	0.084	0.160	0.204	0.243	0.287	0.316	0.343	0.376	0.399
67	0.084	0.158	0.203	0.241	0.284	0.314	0.341	0.373	0.396
68	0.083	0.157	0.201	0.239	0.282	0.311	0.338	0.370	0.393
69	0.082	0.156	0.200	0.237	0.280	0.309	0.336	0.368	0.390
70	0.082	0.155	0.198	0.235	0.278	0.307	0.333	0.365	0.388

71	0.081	0.154	0.197	0.234	0.276	0.305	0.331	0.363	0.385
72	0.081	0.153	0.195	0.232	0.274	0.303	0.329	0.360	0.382
73	0.080	0.152	0.194	0.230	0.272	0.301	0.327	0.358	0.380
74	0.080	0.151	0.193	0.229	0.271	0.299	0.324	0.355	0.377
75	0.079	0.150	0.191	0.227	0.269	0.297	0.322	0.353	0.375
76	0.078	0.149	0.190	0.226	0.267	0.295	0.320	0.351	0.372
77	0.078	0.148	0.189	0.224	0.265	0.293	0.318	0.349	0.370
78	0.077	0.147	0.188	0.223	0.264	0.291	0.316	0.346	0.368
79	0.077	0.146	0.186	0.221	0.262	0.289	0.314	0.344	0.365
80	0.076	0.145	0.185	0.220	0.260	0.287	0.312	0.342	0.363
81	0.076	0.144	0.184	0.219	0.259	0.285	0.310	0.340	0.361
82	0.075	0.143	0.183	0.217	0.257	0.284	0.308	0.338	0.359
83	0.075	0.142	0.182	0.216	0.255	0.282	0.306	0.336	0.357
84	0.074	0.141	0.181	0.215	0.254	0.280	0.305	0.334	0.355
85	0.074	0.140	0.180	0.213	0.252	0.279	0.303	0.332	0.353
86	0.074	0.139	0.179	0.212	0.251	0.277	0.301	0.330	0.351
87	0.073	0.139	0.177	0.211	0.250	0.276	0.299	0.328	0.349
88	0.073	0.138	0.176	0.210	0.248	0.274	0.298	0.327	0.347
89	0.072	0.137	0.175	0.209	0.247	0.272	0.296	0.325	0.345
90	0.072	0.136	0.174	0.207	0.245	0.271	0.294	0.323	0.343
91	0.072	0.135	0.173	0.206	0.244	0.269	0.293	0.321	0.341
92	0.071	0.135	0.173	0.205	0.243	0.268	0.291	0.319	0.339
93	0.071	0.134	0.172	0.204	0.241	0.267	0.290	0.318	0.338
94	0.070	0.133	0.171	0.203	0.240	0.265	0.288	0.316	0.336
95	0.070	0.133	0.170	0.202	0.239	0.264	0.287	0.314	0.334

Table C. *(Continued)*

$\alpha(2)$:	*0.50*	*0.20*	*0.10*	*0.05*	*0.02*	*0.01*	*0.005*	*0.002*	*0.001*
$\alpha(1)$:	*0.25*	*0.10*	*0.05*	*0.025*	*0.01*	*0.005*	*0.0025*	*0.001*	*0.0005*
n									
96	0.070	0.132	0.169	0.201	0.238	0.262	0.285	0.313	0.332
97	0.069	0.131	0.168	0.200	0.236	0.261	0.284	0.311	0.331
98	0.069	0.130	0.167	0.199	0.235	0.260	0.282	0.310	0.329
99	0.068	0.130	0.166	0.198	0.234	0.258	0.281	0.308	0.327
100	0.068	0.129	0.165	0.197	0.233	0.257	0.279	0.307	0.326

For the table entries through $n = 11$, we used the exact distribution of Σd^2 (Owen, 1962: 400–406). For $n = 12$, the exact distribution of de Jonge and von Montfort (1972) was used; and for n's of 13 through 16, we used the exact distributions of Otten (1973). For larger n, the Pearson curve approximations described by Olds (1938) were employed, the accuracy obtained being discussed elsewhere (Zar, 1972). For n larger than those in this table, we may utilize either Table D.21 or, equivalently, Equation (18.2). The accuracy of this procedure is discussed by Zar (1972).

Table D. The Chi-Squared Distribution

df	$\chi^2_{.005}$	$\chi^2_{.025}$	$\chi^2_{.05}$	$\chi^2_{.90}$	$\chi^2_{.95}$	$\chi^2_{.975}$	$\chi^2_{.99}$	$\chi^2_{.995}$
1	.0000393	.000982	.00393	2.706	3.841	5.024	6.635	7.879
2	.0100	.0506	.103	4.605	5.991	7.378	9.210	10.597
3	0.717	.216	.352	6.251	7.815	9.348	11.345	12.838
4	.207	.484	.711	7.779	9.488	11.143	13.277	14.860
5	.412	.831	1.145	9.236	11.070	12.832	15.086	16.750
6	.676	1.237	1.635	10.645	12.592	14.449	16.812	18.548
7	.989	1.690	2.167	12.017	14.067	16.013	18.475	20.278
8	1.344	2.180	2.733	13.362	15.507	17.535	20.090	21.955
9	1.735	2.700	3.325	14.684	16.919	19.023	21.666	23.589
10	2.156	3.247	3.940	15.987	18.307	20.483	23.209	25.188
11	2.603	3.816	4.575	17.275	19.675	21.920	24.725	26.757
12	3.074	4.404	5.226	18.549	21.026	23.336	26.217	28.300
13	3.565	5.009	5.892	19.812	22.362	24.736	27.688	29.819
14	4.075	5.629	6.571	21.064	23.685	26.119	29.141	31.319
15	4.601	6.262	7.261	22.307	24.996	27.488	30.578	32.801
16	5.142	6.908	7.962	23.542	26.296	28.845	32.000	34.267
17	5.697	7.564	8.672	24.769	27.587	30.191	33.409	35.718
18	6.265	8.231	9.390	25.989	28.869	31.526	34.805	37.156
19	6.844	8.907	10.117	27.204	30.144	32.852	36.191	38.582
20	7.434	9.591	10.851	28.412	31.410	34.170	37.566	39.997
21	8.034	10.283	11.591	29.615	32.671	35.479	38.932	41.401
22	8.643	10.982	12.338	30.813	33.924	36.781	40.289	42.796

Table D. *(Continued)*

df	$\chi^2_{.005}$	$\chi^2_{.025}$	$\chi^2_{.05}$	$\chi^2_{.90}$	$\chi^2_{.95}$	$\chi^2_{.975}$	$\chi^2_{.99}$	$\chi^2_{.995}$
23	9.260	11.688	13.091	32.007	35.172	38.076	41.638	44.181
24	9.886	12.401	13.848	33.196	36.415	39.364	42.980	45.558
25	10.520	13.120	14.611	34.382	37.652	40.646	44.314	46.928
26	11.160	13.844	15.379	35.563	38.885	41.923	45.642	48.290
27	11.808	14.573	16.151	36.741	40.113	43.194	46.963	49.645
28	12.461	15.308	16.928	37.916	41.337	44.461	48.278	50.993
29	13.121	16.047	17.708	39.087	42.557	45.722	49.588	52.336
30	13.787	16.791	18.493	40.256	43.773	46.979	50.892	53.672
35	17.192	20.569	22.465	46.059	49.802	53.203	57.342	60.275
40	20.707	24.433	26.509	51.805	55.758	59.342	63.691	66.766
45	24.311	28.366	30.612	57.505	61.656	65.410	69.957	73.166
50	27.991	32.357	34.764	63.167	67.505	71.420	76.154	79.490
60	35.535	40.482	43.188	74.397	79.082	83.298	88.379	91.952
70	43.275	48.758	51.739	85.527	90.531	95.023	100.425	104.215
80	51.172	57.153	60.391	96.578	101.879	106.629	112.329	116.321
90	59.196	65.647	69.126	107.565	113.145	118.136	124.116	128.299
100	67.328	74.222	77.929	118.498	124.342	129.561	135.807	140.169

SOURCE: A. Hald & S.A. Sinkback, *Skandinavisk Aktuarietidskrift, 33,* 1950. Reprinted with permission from Skandinavisk Aktuarietidskrift.

Author Index

Page numbers in *italics* refer to reference pages.

Bestor, D. K., 295, *299*

Subject Index